VIRUS

VIRUS

Vaccinations, the CDC, and the Hijacking of America's Response to the Pandemic

UPDATED AND REVISED

NINA BURLEIGH

Seven Stories Press
New York • Oakland • London

Seven Stories Press
140 Watts Street
New York, NY 10013
www.sevenstories.com

College professors and high school and middle school teachers may order free examination copies of Seven Stories Press titles. Visit https://www.sevenstories.com/pg/resources-academics or email academics@sevenstories.com.

Library of Congress Cataloging-in-Publication Data

Names: Burleigh, Nina, author.
Title: Virus : vaccinations, the CDC, and the hijacking of America's response to the pandemic / Nina Burleigh.
Description: New York, NY : Seven Stories Press, [2021]
Identifiers: LCCN 2021012508 (print) | LCCN 2021012509 (ebook) | ISBN 9781644211809 (hardcover) | ISBN 9781644212004 (paperback) | ISBN 9781644211816 (ebook)
Subjects: LCSH: COVID-19 Pandemic, 2020---United States. | Epidemics--United States--History--21st century. | Denialism. | Vaccines--Social aspects.
Classification: LCC RA644.C67 B873 2021 (print) | LCC RA644.C67 (ebook) | DDC 614.5/92414--dc23
LC record available at https://lccn.loc.gov/2021012508
LC ebook record available at https://lccn.loc.gov/2021012509

Printed in the USA

9 8 7 6 5 4 3 2 1

CONTENTS

PREFACE

One of my first instincts in the surreal early days of lockdown in March 2020 was to hunt down my dog-eared, yellowed, graduate school paperback copy of Daniel Defoe's *A Journal of the Plague Year*. Glued to it for long hours that week, and returning to it occasionally over the course of the past year, I kept being struck by how little has changed in the three and a half centuries since the epidemic that decimated London in the 1660s. Everything, from the nature of and response to the early rumors to the growing sense of unease and the closing of houses of entertainment, from the quack cures and conspiracy theories to the rich fleeing the city and the poor dying in it, from mental health breaking down and mad, cooped-up people breaking free of quarantine and roaming the streets in violation of curfews and sanitary rules—all of it. Just like us. How little the human race has changed since those days without plumbing, electricity, jets, or antibiotics.

And yet, of course, we have evolved in one very significant way: unlike those poor Londoners and every other human being on earth faced with infectious disease epidemics since before recorded history, in 2020 we—the whole planet—knew exactly what was stalking us within weeks of the first deaths: a spiked-protein microbial pathogen. And we had the means, thanks to advances in scientific understanding in the last century and a half, and especially to leaps made in the first two decades of the twenty-first century, to fight back in an array of ways, and then to (hopefully) close this chapter with new vaccines produced in record time.

My aim in this book is simple: to record how we responded to this pandemic, as a society and scientifically, so that we will be sure to do better the next time. More pathogens are on their way, probably at an increased rate, as I explain in chapter 5. We have the means to fight back with a power unlike what any of our ancestors could bring to bear. But are we on a path to avoid half a million American dead—or more—the next time around?

The chaotic sequence of events that began in January 2020 and which continues to unfold today has been so unlike anything we as a society had ever experienced, so tragic, so disorienting, that it has been nearly impossible to absorb and make sense of the whole of it. Especially in the early months, when we were told to stock up and shelter, and as the first wave of death slammed New York, our state of shock distracted us from keeping track of what our leaders were doing. Grave— one could say criminal—decisions and mistakes were made. The American habit of forgetting our defeats is ingrained in us, as medical anthropologist Martha Louise Lincoln, whom I quote in chapter 5, explains.

Because I've spent chunks of my career covering American politics, including, for the last five years, the Trump administration, I have a strong foundational understanding of the ideological and political framework within which decisions get made in American government, including the religious and financial poles of power in which the pandemic response was hatched. But in real time no one journalist or team of journalists could have synthesized all the moving parts and come away saying: *This is how it happened.*

In order to write this book, I have tried to take a broad and balanced view of the pandemic response in government, in politics, and in culture. I studied granular reporting from inside US hospitals and reports issued by the WHO; I looked at what was happening at food banks and at local public health agencies. I watched the changes over the course of the year at the White House, at federal agencies in Washington, and at the great labs in Cambridge and Palo Alto and Bethesda. I also dipped into the fact-challenged universe of Fox News and YouTube and Reddit, because on another plane these places were also where America's response to the pandemic was being shaped. I scoured hundreds of pieces of daily journalism and relied on some terrific investigative reporting, especially by Ed Yong in the *Atlantic*, and the teams at the *New York Times* and at ProPublica, and Katherine Eban in *Vanity Fair*.

I read a variety of books about the current state of American politics and political culture, the most significant being Jane Mayer's *Dark Money*, Greg Grandin's *The End of the Myth*, and Shoshana Zuboff's *The Age of Surveillance Capitalism*. Needless to say, we need both the daily reporting and the longer, more considered analysis that can only happen in books.

And I questioned myself, my assumptions, my fears and hopes. I could not have written this book had I thought I already knew most of the answers when I started.

A year ago, as the first edition of this book was published, I wore green, the color of renewal, to talk to a Zoom audience. Compared with the preceding year, it was a rather merry month of May. Sixty-five percent of Americans had been vaccinated at least once and many were lining up to get their second shots. The Biden administration had mustered the full force of the federal government to get vaccinations into arms, tens of millions of deep-frozen doses to vaccination centers. The elderly and immunocompromised were already vaccinated, so were the frontline workers and teachers who would take it, and now, everyone who wanted the vaccine could get one at a stadium or local pharmacy. The new president had even installed a real scientist inside the White House, filling a job the former administration had left vacant (leaving more room for evangelical counselors and their weekly cabinet prayer meetings). The new science adviser understood the novel language of genetics, the science behind the best of the vaccines.

It looked for a moment like science was winning.

But then, nothing went the way we hoped it would. The wave of antivaccination fervor had started small, but by late summer was swamping whole communities. Pastors and Republicans alike boarded the Good Ship Bullshit to ride it out. The unvaccinated proceeded to overwhelm hospitals as two Covid variants in succession surged across the country.

By winter 2022, even Dr. Fauci was conceding that a hard core of resisters was beyond persuasion. By then, the top government virologist had grown accustomed to death threats against himself and his family. And the White House scientist? He was forced to resign after less than a year, for "bullying and demeaning his subordinates."

Another pandemic year has passed since science tossed humanity the life preserver of the vaccine. The mRNA platform, product of decades of research in genetic medicine, much of it conducted in America by American researchers and in the end funded by American taxpayers, did not, in fact, save children from another year of disrupted education, or restore the near-broken health care system to something like normal routine.

No. Instead, American exceptionalism looks like this: we are about to pass one million dead as I write these words. We lead the developed world in Covid deaths.

Commentators stopped comparing the Covid number to Americans lost in wars a while ago, but by the spring of 2022 about as many of us will have died of Covid as in the nation's two deadliest conflicts combined—World War II and the Civil War.

More Americans have already died of Covid than died of the Spanish flu pandemic—a virus that ravaged the nation a hundred years ago, before jets, the space age, antibiotics, and before the molecular medicine that produced the mRNA vaccine was even a gleam in any scientist's eye.

A few months before Covid swept through Wuhan in late 2019, the United States was the nation deemed most likely to weather a pandemic. Among European nations, only the poorer ones, Russia, Czech Republic, Poland—nations without access to the vaccines available to us—had higher death rates than America's this winter.

I propose three exceptionally American reasons for this:

Greed, having too much of everything except what's good for us, and what we might call our Idiocracy.

Vulture capitalism and related anti-government ideology, plus the need to get reelected, drove the Trump administration's initial response to the virus. A more progressive leadership would certainly have applied the levers of government more effectively and perhaps even leveraged the pandemic to try to make the private health care system more public.

When the virus hit, Americans were already among the unhealthiest people in the developed world. One reason for that is the lack of decent, affordable health care. The other is the *Wall-E* effect of abundance and physical idleness. Covid thrived on our comorbidities.

Finally, Idiocracy ascendant. (If you have not seen the Mike Judge 2006 movie of the same name, do it now. Set five hundred years in the future, it looks almost like a documentary about America today.) Powerful right-wing media machinery has long primed millions to believe that climate change scientists and others ringing alarm bells about industrial waste were tools of the Left and "global elites." Years of fake science to prop up big tobacco and now the fossil fuel industry, plus vulture capitalism, widening wealth inequality, and underfunded public education, have left Americans simultaneously angry, confused about facts, deeply distrustful of experts, and lacking critical thinking skills.

Still, in late spring 2021, Covid death curves were down in some corners of the country. New York City, which had been bleak, apocalyptically vacant, and boarded up post–George Floyd unrest was coming back to life. Musicians played in Washington Square Park and the cloud of cannabis wafting from that ground zero of happiness covered city blocks across Greenwich Village. People went out to eat at the wooden Covid huts on the sidewalks outside Manhattan restaurants. Sex parties surged.

Freed from lockdown, healthy, vaccinated, and restless, I double-masked and went out in the world. I submitted to countless nasal swabs in order to enter and reenter airports and jets, crossing state and national borders. I flew around America, New Mexico, Illinois, and Michigan, and wandered through hamlets and towns.

Then I went abroad. From Paris to Athens, and farther east into Armenia, down into the Caribbean, the scale of the pandemic became more real to me than it had sitting at my desk and scanning the daily *New York Times* pandemic photo montages. Everywhere in the world, men, women, and children are masked up.

To witness this in real life was a powerful and profound reminder that covid is species-wide. The vaccine, on the other hand, is not. It has been free and available to all Americans. It is widely administered in developed countries in Europe. But for the majority of human beings on the African continent and in parts of Asia, the life preserver has been and will remain out of reach.

We have learned to dread disinterred ancient Greek letters—especially the deadly ones Delta and Omicron. Scientists agreed to use the Greek system in order not to tar whole nations as disease incubators—the old way of doing things. The Delta variant emerged in India, Omicron incubated in South Africa—nations teeming with poor, unvaccinated people. The likelihood of this happening was well understood by epidemiologists and virologists. The best way to avert it was equally well known: vaccinate as many human beings on the planet as rapidly as possible to limit the bodies the virus could inhabit, until the pandemic abated.

American taxpayers subsidized the rapid development of the vaccines. Public money—our money—then paid hundreds of millions of dollars to purchase large quantities of the vaccine. The government provided the means to deliver it to now hundreds of millions of Americans.

But even in a global emergency like this one the pharmaceutical industry could not or would not shift its profit-oriented priorities. Taxpayers forked over nearly a billion dollars to Moderna to create the vaccine, and another $4.9 billion to buy three hundred million doses last year. But the company would neither share credit on the patent, nor share the secret recipe with developing nations.

In spring 2021, President Biden signaled his support for waiving patent rights of the vaccine makers, so poor countries could have access to the mRNA formula and make it themselves. The mere whiff of that restriction on the horizon drove share prices lower on Wall Street immediately. Within weeks, Big Pharma was attacking Biden. PhRMA, a lobby group representing some thirty pharmaceutical giants, double-teamed Capitol Hill and blanketed Facebook and Google with a digital ad campaign, to educate the public about "the risks" of patent waiver.

This was all happening as the companies raked in massive and unpredicted profits. The pandemic created a market for Covid-19 vaccines bigger than Wall Street's rosy projections. According to the *Wall Street Journal*, Pfizer and Moderna pulled in a combined $35 billion in Covid-19 vaccine sales globally in the first nine months of 2021. Analysts estimate booster shots will increase sales to a total of $52 billion in 2022.

The patent waiver proposal was DOA, of course. It was never revived, not even after two waves of variants, incubated in poor, unvaccinated parts of the world, forced the heavily vaccinated wealthy nations to backpedal on masks and lockdowns, pushed hospitals to breaking point, and lengthened and worsened global supply chain crises and social upheaval.

Around Christmas '21, as the Omicron variant canceled holiday gatherings and American toy shoppers noticed supply chain disruptions had depleted the customary cornucopia of choice on holiday store shelves, there was a tiny blip of protest from an unusual quarter. Some of Moderna's own stockholders revolted against the company's stand against sharing the technology.

"Instead of being transparent and using its life-saving technology to help curb the pandemic, Moderna is doing the opposite, obfuscating its patent dispute with the US government, ignoring the death and suffering of millions worldwide, and declining to share their technology to help alleviate the stranglehold that COVID-19 has placed on the global economy," said Diana Kearney, senior legal adviser for Legal and Shareholder Advocacy at Oxfam, one of Moderna's shareholders.

The revolt may have had some effect. Quietly in early 2022, Moderna pulled back on its demand that the government be excluded from its vaccine patent. But the world still won't reach the WHO goal of achieving 70 percent vaccine coverage globally by mid-2022.

Whether more and more deadly variants will incubate in unvaccinated people around the world remains to be seen. The only thing certain is that more variants and more waves will probably not change the minds of the anti-vaccine third of Americans. "It's just another variant," Dianne Putnam, an unvaccinated resident of Dalton, Georgia, and president of her county's Republican Party, told the *New York Times* at Christmas. Putnam was sanguine about the virus, although she had spent six days in the hospital after contracting Covid-19. "Next year there'll be another one," she said. "I mean, there's going to always be different variants."

As people like Putnam went about unvaxxed, hospitals were cracking under the strain of trying to save them when they got sick. "Help" ran a full-page ad in the *Cleveland Plain Dealer* in January, paid for by a consortium of area hospitals, Cleveland Clinic, University Hospitals, MetroHealth, Summa Health, Cleveland VA Medical Center, and St. Vincent Charity Medical Center.

America has a habit of "moving on" from its mistakes and failures. The folly of the Iraq War, for example, never received the same kind of comprehensive US public inquiry as it did in the British Chilcot report. The likelihood of anyone in either media or government being held accountable for the cavalier profiteering and science denialism that marked the Trump regime's handling of the pandemic grows dimmer daily.

Many watchdogs in journalism and government are still trying to unravel the Gordian knot of sketchy contracting, alleged fraud, and callous political decision making. Besides excellent investigative journalism from outlets like ProPublica and the *New York Times*, the General Accounting Office (GAO) and the Pandemic Response Accountability Committee (PRAC) are still studying government contracts and looking for fraud among recipients of federal Covid relief funds. PRAC's work has led to criminal charges against hundreds of accused citizen relief fund fraudsters. The GAO reports continue to point out ways agencies could have done better.

The politicization of the pandemic is another challenge altogether. In Congress, the House select subcommittee on the coronavirus crisis, established in April 2020, is doggedly pursuing leads, subpoenaing people and documents. Its work is eclipsed by investigations into the January 6 fascist uprising. It will certainly be disbanded as soon as Republicans retake the House.

In its year-end report the subcommittee revealed details of the concerted effort at the Trump White House to lie about the risks of the virus. The subcommittee announced it had "obtained evidence detailing attempts by Trump White House officials and political appointees to block CDC scientists from speaking to the public for the first three months of the pandemic; to alter or block at least 12 public health guidelines drafted by CDC scientists from being released to the public; to pressure CDC scientists to adopt the Trump administration's policy positions and talking points even when they conflicted with science; and to make changes to at least 13 Morbidity and Mortality Weekly Reports (MMWR) related to the pandemic."

These things were hardly news to people who had paid attention. We watched it happen in real time. But truth, as we now must accept, is malleable. The Covid infodemic had deadly consequences. But if courts and law enforcement agencies can't get the conspiracists of the extreme Right for inciting a deadly, televised insurrection, or get Donald Trump for trading weapons for political dirt on opponents, or for violating the Hatch Act or for rape or for ignoring the Presidential Records Act, what entity can we expect to hold anyone accountable for lies leading to, now, a million mostly preventable American deaths?

There were no laws against it.

ACKNOWLEDGMENTS

I am grateful to the following people: Dan Simon for suggesting and editing this project; Vivian Zhong for schooling me on the science and for being an all-around sounding board. I also want to shout out my thanks to the rest of the Seven Stories team, especially Lauren Hooker, Jon Gilbert, Susan Steiger, Bill Rusin, and Ruth Weiner. I also want to thank Grey Puett for his deep dive into internet conspiracy theories. I very much appreciate the time and thoughts of Dr. Paul Offit, Robert Langer, Dr. Bruce Y. Lee, Dr. David Relman, Martha Louise Lincoln, Jessica Malaty Rivera, and Missy Peña. The work of the CDC investigative team at ProPublica and the pandemic health agency reporting in the *New York Times* were indispensable. Also: Stephanie Slewka, Ianthe Dugan, Jamie Gordon, Matthew Grace, Jason Baruch, Jay Kelly for providing the wood stove in the writer shack, Erik and Felix Freeland for wood-chopping.

CHAPTER I

Smash the State

*I'd actually like to go back to the old times
of Tudor England. I'd put the heads on pikes, right? I'd put
them at the two corners of the White House as a warning
to federal bureaucrats: You either get with
the program or you're gone.*

—STEVE BANNON,

urging the beheading of Dr. Anthony Fauci

There are many ways to begin to tell the story of why more Americans died of Covid-19, the disease caused by SARS-CoV-2, than in any other nation on earth. We could start at the Washington, DC, hospital with doctors amputating the lower leg of the White House chief of security, a man who caught Covid in Donald Trump's mask-free domain. Or we could talk to the families of forty-six veterans who died within days of each other in a Veterans Administration nursing home in Alabama. Or we could listen in on a therapy session with some of the New York City medics struggling with PTSD after helplessly watching some of tens of thousands of people die in a matter of weeks.

Since this story involves mass death, religious zealots, and the worst case of government malpractice in the history of the United States, I'll choose the biblical opening:

In the beginning, there was the State.
And the ideologues said, Let It Be Smashed.
And so it was smashed.

ATLANTA

March 6. Centers for Disease Control.

Early days in the shit show.

Cameras are rolling. The journalists are penned off like lab monkeys awaiting morsels of information about an increasingly confusing government response to an unprecedented crisis.

A plague visits the planet. Not the long-expected brain-eating zombie plague. Another one. A virus that starts out feeling like a common cold then coagulates blood and make lungs look like "ground glass" on X-rays. Starves people of oxygen—sometimes before they even notice.

Americans are just starting to die. Infested cruise ships are stranded in ports around the world. No one has yet decided what to do—or if they have to do anything.

Nobody in this great edifice of American public health—the *gold standard* for the whole world, journalists will write and write again—is yet wearing a mask.

The president of the United States of America is the emcee, clad in the casual costume he wears for events slightly more important than golfing but less serious than his official duties—including hustling foreign leaders and rousing the rabble at rallies. He's zipped his White House bomber jacket (retails for $122 at the White House Gift Shop, presidential seal above left breast) over his gut. The effect is convex, truly bomb-like, containing the protuberance. Below that, a pair of khakis. White dress shirt. Red MAGA hat, brim cocked level just above the raccoon white circles around his eyes.

The set for this show is a real lab. A table is laden with dozens of very large hand-pump sanitizer bottles. There's a shortage of this stuff around the country right now—one more small crazy fact that is freaking Americans out—but there's plenty of it here by the president. The president will gesture at the bottles and remind the assembled that he never liked to shake hands anyway and certainly doesn't press the flesh as a politician—something, he is careful to add, most politicians do but which is one of the myriad things that sets him apart from that odious herd.

The other three men are more formal, as befits their position, hosts of this auspicious public health event with the leader of the free world. They wear suits and ties. Two of them have advanced medical degrees, one is a lawyer and political appointee. They stand beside a man who has spewed going on sixteen thousand lies to the American public through the biggest bullhorn on the planet. The sensation of his nearness affects them differently, on a spectrum from self-conscious embarrassment, to toady awe in the presence of greatness, to barely veiled terror.

Health and Human Service (HHS) secretary Alex Azar, trim, bearded, a lawyer by training with no medical experience other than as a Big Pharma exec, gazes up at his boss with the eyes of a Labrador at heel; Centers for Disease Control (CDC) director Dr. Robert Redfield, whose white chin and side whiskers are trimmed in the fashion of a nineteenth-century vicar, can barely contain the fulsome gratitude he will shortly pour on the red-hatted head. "Well, I think I—first, I want to thank you for your decisive leadership in helping us, you know, put public health first," he says. "I also want to thank you for coming here today and—and sort of encouraging and bringing energy to the men and women that you see that work every day to try to keep America safe. So I think that's the most important thing I want to say, sir."

A man named Dr. Steve Monroe, colorless and quivering, stands by. He is the guy who, this morning, has drawn the short straw or, actually, the hara-kiri knife of explaining to the media just what the hell is going on with the strange, slow rollout of the CDC's Covid tests.

In New York City, frontline nurses and doctors were about to be overwhelmed with a wave of people turning blue from lack of oxygen in their blood, whose legs were mysteriously filling with clots and going black. Twenty thousand people would die while doctors tried to understand what drugs or procedures might mitigate the strange constellation of Covid symptoms. Victims endured horrible final days connected to ventilators. Their blood gelled in their veins. Their organs failed one by one within hours.

No one knows how bad it's going to get. But it is impossible to look at footage of the scene now without an uncanny shiver. The room behind the men is white, lab-white, festooned with black wires dangling above desktop computers. Georgia senator Kelly Loeffler—fresh off allegations that she did some insider trading off the pandemic briefing she received before the market crashed—and governor Brian Kemp are there too, notching a photo op with the big guy.

Dr. Monroe is up first. There's been a bit of a problem with the tests, he avers, without addressing the elephant in the room, the major discrepancies between Trump saying "anyone who wants a test can get one" and Azar claiming "four million tests will be available by the end of next week" and what the CDC's star virus hunter Anne Schuchat (played by Kate

Winslet in the 2011 movie *Contagion*) has just told Congress: that the CDC has conducted only three thousand tests on five hundred people.

Five hundred people, in a nation of three hundred million, was hardly the same as "anybody who wants a test can get tested."

Dr. Monroe's queasy mien, then. He looks like he would rather be anywhere but in front of a media gaggle, with a red-MAGA-hatted giant looming over him, officiously interjecting periodically to ask reporters, "Did you understand that?"

"In this laboratory is where we generate materials that go into all of our diagnostic tests, not just for the coronavirus, which you have the electron micrograph here, but also for all of the other infectious agents that we work with," Dr. Monroe starts, in a monotone. "And the advantage of having this facility here is the CDC is constantly listening for infectious disease spreads, both within the US and around the world. And when we first heard about this unusual illness in Wuhan, China, we started paying close attention to see if there was any indication of what might be the cause. And as soon as the Chinese announced that it was a coronavirus and made available to the general public the sequence of that virus, we immediately started using that information—our scientists—to develop a test so that we could detect the virus. . . . And so, we worked with the FDA to get—"

Trump interrupts: "So tell them about how you've done with the tests [inaudible] over four million."

Dr. Monroe: "—to get what we call 'emergency use authorization.'"

Dr. Monroe knows what no one in the media arrayed before him understands—but which Azar, Dr. Redfield, and Trump do: no mass Covid testing for Americans anytime soon—if ever.

They throw it to the media. First question: What about that infested cruise ship?

San Francisco won't let a cruise ship with dozens of infected passengers, the *Grand Princess*, dock. Passengers are frantic, locked in their cabins, FaceTiming their terror onto social media. *Help us!*

The president announces he isn't going to intervene with San Francisco. "I like the numbers being where they are," he says. "I don't need to have the numbers double because of one ship. That wasn't our fault."

Journalist: "Obviously, Mr. President, we've talked a lot about the health ramifications, which of course is very important. But there are also economic ramifications; the stock market dropped again today. The travel industry—airlines, cruise ships, other companies—travel companies have been hit especially hard. Can you give us a sense of what you're considering to help offset this pain?"

Trump: "Well, we're considering different things. But we're also considering the fact that last year we had approximately thirty-six thousand deaths due to what's called the flu. And I was—when I first heard this four, five, six weeks ago—when I was hearing the amount of people that died with flu, I was shocked to hear it. Anywhere from twenty-seven thousand to seventy thousand or seventy-seven thousand. And I guess they said, in 1990, that was in particular very bad; it was higher than that. As of the time I left the plane with you, we had two hundred and forty cases. That's at least what was on a very fine network known as Fox News. And you love it. But that's what I happened to be watching. And how was the show last night? Did it get good ratings, by the way?"

Journalist: "I—I don't know, sir."

Trump: "Oh, really? I heard it broke all ratings records, but maybe that's wrong. That's what they told me. I don't know. I can't imagine that."

Trump will maintain focus on the flu: "When people have the flu, you have an average of thirty-six thousand people dying. I've never heard those numbers. I would—I would've been shocked. I would've said, 'Does anybody die from the flu?' I didn't know people died from the flu—thirty-six thousand people died."

Azar and Dr. Redfield maintain poker faces. Dr. Monroe is ashen.

Fact check: Trump in that moment knows the flu kills people. It's family lore, how his grandfather dropped dead of it in 1919, leaving a German-speaking widow with three kids to found a small building company in Queens, a death that forever altered the trajectory of the Trump clan. He knows the virus is worse than the flu. He's said as much to Bob Woodward: "Much, much more deadly."

But he's on his way to clocking sixteen thousand lies to the American public in his official capacity. Like all the others, this one rolling off his tongue in a syrupy Rat Pack croon.

DOCTOR WHO?

No one had done four million "perfect" Covid tests in America as of March 6. Trump just tossed that number out, made it up out of thin air in order to interrupt Dr. Monroe before Dr. Monroe could explain that the Food and Drug Administration (FDA) needs to give its tests special authorization because, far from perfect, they are flawed.

The US government could have accepted tests developed by the World Health Organization (WHO) as early as February.

The FDA could have, on an emergency basis, allowed commercial test makers to make and distribute some. The FDA's failure to urgently adjust rules on an emergency basis in the testing case could be chalked up to the logjams of bureaucracy. But that bureaucracy could and would act fast when Trump ordered it to get behind a malaria drug as an unproven Covid cure.

The slow-walked tests were no accident. The Chinese shared a new disease's genome with the world on January 11, and within days the WHO developed a rapid test for it and offered it to the world. American infectious disease experts were already alarmed in mid-January, but the Trump regime declined to use it when offered in February.

He liked the numbers low.

But also, ideology: the Trump regime came to power nose-snubbing the international community, especially the United Nations, run by bureaucrats with unpronounceable names from the Global South that spurned Israel, sucked up American aid, and yet failed to recognize American greatness. For the audience at home, the base, a key element in shrinking and decentralizing government was removing the United States from world organizations like the United Nations, which right-wingers had long suspected was inching ever closer to forcing us to accept a dangerously unified globe without national borders.

Trump was down with that. He had already pulled the United States out of UNESCO, the cultural arm of the United Nations, in 2017, followed by the UNHCR, the UN's refugee agency. So of course, Trump had declined the offer of tests from the WHO—a member organization, like the United Nations, that the United States joined after World War II.

Screw the WHO and screw your tests. We can do it better.

That decision was, in some ways, the original sin of the pandemic.

It took another month, until early February, for the CDC to craft and send out its tests. Almost immediately, health labs across the country reported a small mistake in the CDC test results. The fix delayed US testing for six more weeks—an eon in virus time. By the time the American government authorized its own test, Covid was rampant, unchecked, spreading human to human in communities, in New York and Seattle and unknown points in between.

It would be impossible to trace or cap.

The story of the CDC test mistake is still subject to dissent. One explanation is that the test kept returning false positives. The other explanation is that a component that tested for flu malfunctioned, and then, in theory, the FDA could have issued an emergency authorization exemption to its rules, allowing labs to use the CDC test anyway. But nobody—least of all the man with the ultimate executive authority—demanded that.

He liked the numbers low.

THE GOLD STANDARD IN GLOBAL PUBLIC HEALTH

The CDC was good at many things. Sending teams to Borneo and Congo to flush out deadly parasites. Stopping Ebola. Vaccinating children. Collecting statistics on Zika and AIDS and cancer clusters and the numbers of American babies with malnutrition.

But it turned out to be helpless against ruthless political leadership. Its leaders would never roll their eyes or stifle a gag when the president started bragging about his Fox ratings or advising Americans to inject bleach. A single contradictory remark could mean a raging tweet, personal doxing, and death threats.

The first person to speak the truth publicly about the pandemic was Dr. Nancy Messonnier, the director of the CDC's

National Center for Immunization and Respiratory Diseases. She caused a stock-market rout when she announced she was preparing her kids for school closures. The president, after hearing about Dr. Messonnier's message on Air Force One, flying back from India where among other adulations he had been feted at a Hindu nationalist rally, tweeted at her by name and threatened to fire her.

The men and women of the CDC and HHS know they are standing on the edge of a cliff. They also know they are trailing after a malignant clown. But the malignant clown serves a very important purpose for some very important men. While this pandemic was not exactly part of the plan, it will serve its implementation.

On July 1, 1946, when the national Communicable Disease Center (it would be renamed in 1970) first opened its doors and occupied one floor of a small building in Atlanta, the United States was coming out of a world war and the Depression, and there was general agreement that government could be a force for good. The CDC's primary mission was to prevent the spread of malaria—still a worry in the swamps and electricity-less backwoods of America as far north as New Jersey. Four hundred employees worked with a budget of $10 million to purchase trucks, sprayers, shovels, and labor to eradicate disease-carrying mosquitoes.

CDC founder Dr. Joseph Mountin grew the small agency over a decade into one that would deserve credit for eradicating many communicable scourges, from polio and parasites to STDs, and providing practical help to state health departments. As the CDC grew, its scientists and medics set up teams around the country and the world to monitor staph outbreaks in hospitals, establish tuberculosis programs, and oversee vaccination programs aimed at polio, measles, mumps, and other childhood diseases.

By the late 1950s, the CDC was becoming the global model of excellence for public health. Its teams were monitoring disease outbreaks and promoting vaccination campaigns around the world. Its elite Epidemic Intelligence Service of globe-trotting disease fighters eventually played a role in eradicating smallpox worldwide, containing Ebola, and performing countless lesser-known missions.

Before the pandemic, America's CDC was the agency other nations looked to for advice and assistance. The Chinese so revered it that they named their own national public health agency after it.

At home, though, the CDC was not so popular.

First, for the hard right, what was "public health," anyway, but socialism?

Second, the CDC was a government agency staffed by elite scientists who infected it with their liberalism and nosed into people's private decisions. Like how to keep teen girls from getting pregnant and what to feed kids. Remember when it developed a healthy curriculum for schools? Ketchup, as Reagan would say, was a fine vegetable for poor kids to eat.

Third, the agency also collected data that put it at cross-purposes with industry. Some of that data collection provoked outright political battles. Congress had had to step in and stop the CDC's federal gun-violence studies, for example. Tobacco didn't cause lung cancer, despite what the scientists at the CDC might think they knew. Since the 1970s, the agency had been a thorn in the side of industry, along with the Occupational Safety and Health Administration, tracking the health effects of environmental degradation from industrial chemicals. The CDC studied cancer clusters in Louisville related to vinyl chloride, and lead poisoning connected to an ore smelter in El Paso.

Finally, the CDC was everything evangelical Christian fanatics wanted to root out. The agency took a common-sense approach to reproductive health and sex education. Its funding of sex-practices studies and its website that included references to the sex practices of teens seemed pro-choice or at least pro-contraception. Its work in the world of sexually transmitted diseases—as well as, eventually, its alliance with Planned Parenthood—sometimes brought it onto the battle-field of the culture wars. Its website was revised on the subject of abortion and contraceptives every time the occupant of the White House changed parties.

Then came AIDS, which initially struck gay men, putting male-to-male anal sex in the scientific and media spotlight. Many of the senior US public health officials facing the 2020 pandemic forged careers during the AIDS epidemic of the late 1980s and 1990s. Dr. Anthony Fauci, the elfin face of scientific reason howling into the wind of Trumpian disinformation, got his start in public health during the AIDS epidemic. Dr. Fauci, with his undergraduate degree in classics, and his non-political post at the helm of the National Institute of Allergy and Infectious Diseases since 1984, would turn out to have the moral backbone and civil-service protection to be able to stand up to Trump. He joined Supreme Court justice Ruth Bader Ginsburg as one of the Trump #resistance geriatric heroes.

The other two scientific leaders of the Trump regime's Covid team also came into public health fighting AIDS—but their fervor was moral as well as scientific. Dr. Robert Redfield and Dr. Deborah Birx are both evangelical Christians whose entries into public health coincided with the AIDS epidemic. Both have been aligned with homophobic organizations. Both were in the Trump administration precisely because those bona fides were more payback to his white evangelical base.

THE IDES OF MARCH

Even before Trump announced he liked the numbers low, members of the pandemic-preparedness community—scientists, medics, policy planners outside the government who studied and made policy recommendations for just such emergencies—were growing more alarmed.

No one could yet quite believe the federal government of the United States was standing down in the hour of the nation's greatest need.

One of those in shock was health-systems expert Dr. Bruce Y. Lee, a CUNY professor and analyst. "In March, people in the community were clamoring, *Do something*," he said. "They were clamoring all over the place, on social media. Public health experts were saying, publicly, *Do this. This is what you should do.* And the response from the White House and from the administration was actually not to do anything. . . . The messaging wasn't there; instead, there's this mixed messaging, talking about how, *Oh, maybe this may go away*, or, *We're rounding the corner*, or whatever synonym you want to have of that statement. Rounding the corner. I never want to say one hundred percent, but I can't think of a single public health expert or infectious disease expert who believed that we were rounding the corner in March. It was quite the opposite. Most everyone that I talked to agreed that we were only at the beginning of a huge problem."

The CDC, when it worked, functioned as a kind of nexus for experts, especially in pandemic preparedness. As awareness of the scale of the challenge grew in February and early March, the pandemic-preparedness community was buzzing with alarm, sharing data and information. It amounted to a massive human resource waiting to be tapped.

But no one from the federal government reached out. And none of them knew whom to call on the inside.

In 2018, under Trump's national security adviser, John Bolton, an Obama-era pandemic-preparedness council at the National Security Council (formed after the Ebola scare in 2014) was disbanded. And the administration had sacked or failed to rehire previous points of contact.

So no one in the pandemic-preparedness community even knew who in the administration *needed* their advice.

When it became clear that the Trump regime would maintain its ideological "small government" course during this time of increasing need, the Rockefeller Foundation in April submitted a detailed plan with the goal of conducting thirty million tests per week by fall 2020 and forming a contact-tracing "health corps" of up to three hundred thousand people. The plan would have brought together a massive coalition of federal agencies, state and local governments, and academics, at a cost of $100 billion.

The Trump administration wasn't interested—no explanation given.

We can assume that such a monumental operation, if successful, might have reinvigorated trust and faith in centralized government and opened a new sector of government assistance and created a new cadre of civil-service workers—all of which were at odds with the goal of promoting a psychology of rugged individualism that spurned the social safety net.

As panic began to spread to American towns and cities, the Rockefeller Foundation was nearly alone in assisting school districts and Native reservations—parts of America as left-behind as Africa was when the Rockefeller Foundation worked to eradicate hookworm beginning in the 1920s.

The absence of testing as a concern was soon lost in the panic over a nationwide shortage of personal protective equipment (PPE). The CDC had also seen this coming since at least the 1990s. In 1999, it launched the National Pharmaceutical Stockpile (now the Strategic National Stockpile)—drugs, vaccines, and other medical products and supplies to provide for national emergency health security. Trump's son-in-law and senior adviser Jared Kushner early on announced—baselessly, it turned out—that the Strategic National Stockpile was for federal, not state, use, and its official government webpage was altered to reflect Kushner's statement.

The administration had been testing the limits of executive authority since opening day and was giddy with pure power: any government website could be altered at the whim of a presidential son-in-law without portfolio.

So could medical expertise!

On March 19, Trump began touting the malaria drug hydroxychloroquine as a possible medicine. The Chinese had thrown this drug at severely ill patients, part of their kitchen-sink strategy. And some reports indicated that some people didn't die. That was good enough for Donald. "The nice part is, it's been around for a long time, so we know that if it—if things don't go as planned, it's not going to kill anybody," he said on March 19.

Two days later, the Trump Twitter account spewed this: "HYDROXYCHLOROQUINE & AZITHROMYCIN, taken together, have a real chance to be one of the biggest game changers in the history of medicine. The FDA has moved mountains—Thank You! Hopefully they will BOTH (H works better with A, International Journal of Antimicrobial Agents)."

Three days later, an Arizona man died after ingesting a version of the substance intended for use in his pet fish tank. Four days after that, the FDA issued an emergency use authorization to allow "hydroxychloroquine sulfate and chloroquine phosphate products" donated to the Strategic National Stockpile to be distributed to hospitalized patients with Covid (the same FDA that had dragged its feet on authorizing the CDC tests).

More medical advice was coming from our commander in chief.

On April 23, 2020:

"A question that probably some of you are thinking of if you're totally into that world, which I find to be very interesting. So, supposedly we hit the body with a tremendous, whether it's ultraviolet or just very powerful light, and I think you said that hasn't been checked, but you're going to test it. And then I said supposing you brought the light inside the body, which you can do either through the skin or in some other way. . . . Sounds interesting, right?

"And then I see the disinfectant, where it knocks it out in one minute. And is there a way we can do something like that, by injection inside or almost a cleaning, because you see it gets in the lungs and it does a tremendous number on the lungs, so it'd be interesting to check that, so that you're going to have to use medical doctors with, but it sounds interesting to me. So, we'll see, but the whole concept of the light, the way it kills it in one minute. That's pretty powerful."

No one corrected him. Dr. Birx, standing beside the president, looked pained but held her tongue. Dr. Fauci was the only public scientist who dared correct Trump in real time. He sometimes maneuvered his small frame behind the podium and into TV camera range to contradict him. But he wasn't in the briefing room that day.

For his courage, or gall, in contradicting the president on live TV, Dr. Fauci soon became public enemy number one. Trump's base launched him right up there with Nancy Pelosi as an adversary. For months, the career public health scientist calmly fielded death threats to himself and his family. A few other brave souls stepped up to issue correctives. Dr. Rick Bright, director of the Biomedical Advanced Research and Development Agency (BARDA), who had worked in and out of the CDC since 1998, officially resigned from the National Institutes of Health in October, after speaking out against quack cures and trying to arrange for a national testing infrastructure.

"He can no longer countenance working for an administration that puts politics over science to the great detriment of the American people," Dr. Bright's lawyer announced.

NO LEADERSHIP IS GOOD LEADERSHIP

The pillar of Trump's political power, contrary to popular belief, was not the "deplorable" rabble that—inexplicably in the eyes of coastal elites and progressives—voted against their own interests on things like national health care and taxing the super-rich.

Trump's true backers were crony capitalists and stone-cold Koch-bro antigovernment ideologues. They were flanked by Rapture-ready religious zealots. Between them, the moneyed and the Godly were behind decades of brainwashing radio and social-media propaganda about brown people getting free stuff and feminists and gay people stealing a generation of children from the Christian patriarchy.

The two groups had one thing in common: they wanted to dispense with regulations and experts who told them how to run their businesses; what waste they could dispose of where; what to teach and feed their kids; how to treat their farm animals, crops, and lawns; and where they could ride their ATVs and brandish their firearms. They wanted to lay waste to the nanny state governmental apparatus and replace it with a Hobbesian Utopia/Gilead, where the weak no longer taxed the strong. Let God sort it out.

For this goal, the pandemic was a gift from God.

The hard-right long game had always been about preventing poor people, and more precisely poor *brown* people, from taking free stuff. The philosophy crept close to eugenics: when the poor and frail are aided by government and survive, they weaken the American herd. The true believers were one sliver away from saying publicly that the poor don't really need to learn how to read (a conservative Michigan federal judge, dissenting from a 2020 US Court of Appeals ruling that Detroit schoolchildren have a constitutional right to an education, had nearly stated as much).

The great and strange financier behind Trump during the 2016 election, hedge fund billionaire Robert Mercer, studied for his PhD alongside one of the last American proponents of eugenics in academia, Raymond Cattell. In their ideal world, untaxed wealth would be allowed to grow, with corporations and whole industries operating beyond the intrusions of health and safety inspectors, anti-pollution zealots, tree huggers, lovers of protected snails, etc.

Corporatist libertarians and white evangelical Christians got Trump elected with bold aims: nothing less than the remaking of America into a quantum-age Wild West in which money talks and bullshit walks, women stay home or teeter around on fuck-me shoes, useless animals go extinct, God provides coal and oil for humans to extract, and everyone (supposedly) pulls themselves up by their own bootstraps. In this ideal world, the poor, brown, sick, and weak die off, while the white, wealthy, and healthy survive, ensuring the inherent supremacy of the American gene pool.

The regime would pay back the God squad first by letting them colonize the health and human services agencies, where they could dispense with science and focus on rolling back rights for gay people and women. With the Godly thus occupied, and the agencies' eyes on controlling sex lives, not disease, the regime worked on the main goal: demolishing the state.

The Heritage Foundation, a right-wing think tank lavishly funded by billionaires for decades, had colonized the executive branch upon inauguration. The foundation's worker bees buzzed in, hauling rollies stuffed with policy proposals they'd been shining up during years out of power—aimed at eradicating not just the social safety net but whatever remained within the government of any net's supporters. The never-ending Obamacare repeal effort was the subject of many a Heritage policy paper.

In her book *Dark Money*, Jane Mayer describes how the midwestern oil industry billionaire Koch brothers (whose father built oil refineries for Adolf Hitler) spearheaded this operation. The libertarians had lavished their discretionary extra billions for decades on Washington think tanks that invaded the public sector every time a Republican took the White House.

Their aim looked moderate compared to that of Mercer, the shadowy reactionary funder behind Steve Bannon, President Trump's one-time chief strategist, who wanted the US government "shrunk down to the size of a pinhead" and was especially contemptuous of the social safety net.

"Bob believes that human beings have no inherent value other than how much money they make," Philadelphia billionaire David Magerman, a former hedge fund partner of Mercer, told the *Wall Street Journal.* "A cat has value, he's said, because it provides pleasure to humans. But if someone is on welfare they have negative value. If he earns a thousand times more than a schoolteacher, then he's a thousand times more valuable. He thinks society is upside down—that government helps the weak people get strong, and makes the strong people weak by taking their money away, through taxes."

After Magerman's remarks were published, Mercer fired him. Magerman has sued him over it.

EYES ON GOD

At the White House, there were bigger things to worry about than a virus. It was an election year, and the rampaging bullish stock market was the issue on which Trump was betting his entire reelection. And it was about to go bear. This was the panic he had wanted to avoid when he confessed to Bob Woodward that he didn't want a panic.

The crash began on Monday, March 9. The Dow fell 2,013.76 points that day to 23,851.02—at the time, the Dow's worst single-day point drop in US market history. There would be worse days ahead, as the market plummeted for months. These were bad numbers to the investors, but for millions of working families, it meant job loss, actual hardship.

Within weeks, images of miles-long food lines in California started showing up on TV. Congress scrambled and fought over how much of a safety net the American people might need to get through it and the president signed the first bailout—the CARES Act. A measly $1,200 stimulus check was mailed. People who qualified for unemployment could go online and try to cover their monthly expenses.

The day after the stock market first rolled off the cliff and started its monthslong pandemic downturn, Trump strode into the White House briefing room. *This* was a true emergency. Not the virus, chumps. The money!

He announced that he was taking charge of the virus response, kicking out the agency bureaucrats like the one who had inadvertently hurt the Wall Street numbers. Right there, on the spot, he would be the decider.

He would put Vice President Mike Pence—who was standing by in wax figure mode, nodding obsequiously at the man evangelicals had been comparing to Cyrus, the Old Testament Persian king whom God had chosen to save the Jews—in charge of the White House Coronavirus Task Force.

It was an interesting choice.

Antipathy to science had been Pence's political signature throughout his career in Indiana's congressional delegation and then as governor of the Hoosier State. He did give lip service to health in the sense that his career was based on pushing his sect's moral code on the public through public health agencies and laws.

He was the first congressman to try to defund Planned Parenthood, leading what became the Republican war on women's health clinics. As governor of Indiana, Pence presided over the passage of several draconian anti-abortion laws. Under him, Indiana had put a woman, Purvi Patel, in jail for a miscarriage, and fought in the courts to keep her there for twenty years.

(She was released after being incarcerated for more than two years, after out-of-state lawyers came to her rescue and filed appeals.)

Pence's public health assault wasn't limited to females. During his final year as governor, he had chopped Indiana's spending on public health to $12.40 per person, among the lowest in the nation despite Indiana's high rates of obesity, smoking, and infant mortality. He inadvertently fomented an HIV outbreak when he forced a Planned Parenthood clinic in one of the state's poorest counties to shut down, and refused for months to allow state agencies to mount a clean-needle program when the outbreak started, arguably causing dozens of needless deaths.

Before being whisked back to Washington on the Trump magic carpet in 2016, Pence's parting shot at the reproductive rights of Indiana women was to sign a law requiring funerals for all fetuses, so that a woman who miscarried—even without knowing she was pregnant—might be breaking the law if she didn't formally cremate or bury the tissue.

Handing off management of a serious global pandemic to a religious zealot instead of a scientist might not seem like such a good idea. But it made sense in the Trump administration because his white evangelical supporters were the key to his political survival, and they cared more about controlling people's sex lives than just about anything else.

Before the pandemic, one plausible reason for why the Trump regime had not kept its eye firmly on disease outbreaks was that it had been focusing its public health efforts on abolishing abortion, restricting access to contraception, and cutting ties with Planned Parenthood. The CDC involved itself in tracking changes in sexual habits. It was still surveying teens on sex practices, and even offering online links to Planned Parenthood, which was loathed by the right for providing contraceptives and abortion. The biggest advance Trump touted at HHS before the pandemic was prominently displaying a link on the department's homepage for health workers who felt their "religious liberty" was threatened by aspects of their jobs. Trump's CDC had added a page for teens about "abstinence" and a sexual practice it called "outercourse."

In the White House, he had repaid his base handsomely by putting "Pence's people" in control in health and human services areas—defunding Planned Parenthood, gutting the Affordable Care Act with its hated birth control rule. They retooled public health civil rights offices, which the Obama administration had used to promote LGBT rights, and turned them into offices of "Conscience and Religious Freedom." The HHS "conscience rule" would have protected health care workers who object to performing abortions and sterilizations or treating gay and transgender patients. One of the president's first acts after his inauguration was to reinstate a global gag order preventing foreign aid workers under the US government aegis from discussing abortion.

At the United Nations and the WHO, Trump's representatives worked to pull references to "gender" and "sexual and reproductive health" from international rights documents. The Trump administration threatened to veto a UN resolution aimed at combating rape as a weapon of war because of language providing victims with sexual and reproductive health care. The phrase "sexual and reproductive health" was cut from the final resolution, which a spokesperson for the United Nations Population Fund called "regrettable," adding that "denying survivors access to such services is a human rights violation that can have dire consequences."

HHS secretary Azar was a "cabinet sponsor" of evangelical pastor Ralph Drollinger's Capitol Ministries' weekly Bible study group held inside the White House for senior staff. (Drollinger had endeared himself to Trump early by advising him to run America as a "benevolent dictatorship.") Trump's CDC director, Dr. Robert Redfield (appointed to replace Trump's first choice, a doctor whose investments in tobacco and other sketchy financial deals cost her her job), was a lifelong evangelical Christian who had cut his professional teeth fighting AIDS alongside other evangelicals who were moved as much by homophobic zeal as by Christian mercy. He was famous for having ordered, while in the military, that HIV-positive service members be cordoned off, an arrangement likened to putting the sick in a leper colony.

Dr. Redfield and Dr. Birx had both spent decades in the military, and had done some genuine mitigation work in the AIDS field (Obama had even named Dr. Birx his ambassador at large and US global AIDS coordinator). But both Dr. Birx and Dr. Redfield are scientists whose fundamentalist beliefs steer them toward authoritarianism. Advanced science and medical degrees did not eradicate their conviction that some supernatural *He* is ultimately responsible for the course of human events on earth.

The autocratic *He* in the sky had, for many evangelicals, an earthly analogue in the form of the philandering New York reality show star who improbably became the head of the US government. Dr. Redfield came across on TV and at congressional hearings as a laconic grandpa, but behind the scenes he accommodated the administration's need to tamp down the sense of crisis, when good leadership would have demanded that he prepare the public for the severity of what he knew was coming.

At every step, the CDC leader waffled, allowed lies to go unchecked, even helped hide efforts to cook the data. When scientists concluded that the virus was highly contagious and airborne, the CDC released that information along with specifically dangerous places and activities. After White House threats, the agency removed warnings about singing in church. Religious gatherings of all sorts, including at Christian churches on Sunday, continued to be superspreader events for months—and in fact still are as of this writing.

PER OCCASIONEM CHAO*

The virus spread invisibly, unchecked by tests. A little fever here, a dry cough there, a whopping headache, and then wham, sirens all day and all night, gurneys lined up like train cars in New York hospital hallways with supine, gasping people. The truth of this defied the president's repeated claims—now made nightly at increasingly combative press conferences with him at the podium batting away health officials who dared disagree with him—that "everyone who wants [a test] can get one."

By March 11, as a first surge hit emergency rooms, New York City closed its schools, forcing millions of parents to stay home with their children, and further eroding markets. A few weeks later, as the president declared the crisis "totally under control," New York City moved refrigerated trucks to the loading docks of hospitals, and iPhones recorded forklifts moving corpses into them. By April, in an unforgettable scene more reminiscent of Bangladesh after a cyclone than anything ever seen in America's greatest metropolis, contract workers in New York were photographed digging massive trenches in the potter's field on the Bronx's Hart Island for the overflow of human bodies.

---

* In chaos, opportunity.

New Yorkers would die as medical workers went on TV, begging for protective equipment, some in tears, wearing black garbage bags and using the same mask all day. Nurses started showing up sick, then on ventilators, then some were dead.

Meanwhile, public officials across the country—but especially in the New York City metro area, where twenty million people were about to be slammed with a tsunami of death—were suddenly forced to contend with an experiment in chaos capitalism, organized under the leadership of Trump's boy wonder, Jared Kushner.

As the world watched in horror the video of corpses being loaded onto refrigerated trucks in New York, a faction of the Trump regime's inner circle was lifting its head, blinking its yellow eyes, and sniffing the air. This bloc of Trumpworld, inside and outside the administration, recognized the pandemic not for what it took away—human lives, livelihoods—but for what it offered.

The pandemic was actually a fortuitous moment. It was going to make some people very, very rich. They would find opportunity in chaos, fling taxpayer money at private enterprise, enrich already rich friends. Since it was an emergency, and speed was essential, they could dispense with the oversight of government contract officers, federal codes, regulations, procurement databases—all that government muck that hindered the doing of business and the making of money.

The only code they needed were the two letters *WH*.

In *The Shock Doctrine*, Naomi Klein wrote that a strategy of late-stage capitalism is to use—or if not available, create and then use—chaos to give the free market a reboot. The best-known example of this before the pandemic was in the lead-up to the Iraq War, when Dick Cheney was divvying up rights to the oil fields before the bombs fell on Baghdad.

The chaos playbook is simple, but it requires certain pre-conditions. Besides a disaster, it needs blind or nonexistent oversight. The Trump regime provided this in the form of no-bid contracts to a small group of large health care suppliers, let them determine distribution, and brought on MBA mini-me "volunteers" to supposedly coordinate this effort.

This particular chaos allowed them to road-test their dream system—to prove once and for all that the forces of supply and demand, the instinct to make a buck, could do a better job managing a natural disaster than the government and its bureaucrats. With Trump in charge, and already three years into laying waste to the agencies, they could sideline government emergency management experts, put twentysomething kids in charge of distribution, and circulate lists of possible suppliers, one of whom, a Silicon Valley entrepreneur with no medical contracting experience, snagged a cool $86 million contract from the state of New York for ventilators he would never deliver.

Democrats and civil society groups in Washington have filed requests for more information about how those lists were compiled, who got the money, and where the supplies actually went. It is possible we may never know.

In mid-March, an assistant professor of science and technology policy at the Massachusetts Institute of Technology and a member of the Covid-19 Policy Alliance pitched an idea. The government could address the testing and personal protective equipment (PPE) shortage by deploying planes abroad to fetch and deliver loads of needed equipment from source countries. The proposal suggested that once the material was delivered to US hubs, the Covid-19 Policy Alliance would, based on its data, direct it to areas where it was scarce.

The Trump White House, with Kushner at the helm, liked the idea of the planes—but not so much the idea of having a set of data analysts figure out where and how to distribute PPE. Putting financially disinterested experts in charge didn't mesh with their market ideology. Instead, the White House decided that the private sector—specifically, six handpicked health supply giants—could move the supplies faster. Motivated not by altruism, but by profit.

This was the genesis of Project Airbridge, a plan designed to take advantage of the buyer-seller relationships maintained by the largest health industry suppliers in the United States. Soon Trump was braying about it and the White House PR machine was churning out colorful pictures of American planes engaged in a cross between the Berlin airlift and the Apollo moon shot.

At an April 7 White House briefing, while New York governor Andrew Cuomo was frantically trying—without federal assistance—to scramble up ventilators and PPE for overwhelmed city hospitals, and realizing along with other governors that the feds were not going to help, Trump made an announcement. "Through Project Airbridge, we have succeeded in bringing planeloads of vital supplies into the United States from overseas," he said. "These are massive planes, by the way. The big planes—they are very big, very powerful—and they are loaded to the gills with supplies."

A month later, in May, the White House press secretary, Kayleigh McEnany, stood beside a poster emblazoned with the number 720,000—supposedly the number of miles that one hundred Project Airbridge flights had covered. The poster trumpeted that the distance was "More than 3 trips to the moon!" McEnany claimed the flights had delivered "nearly one billion pieces" of PPE to hospitals and areas in need.

Journalists fact-checked her claims and those of Vice President Pence, who had been crowing that Project Airbridge delivered twenty-two million surgical masks daily. From Federal Emergency Management Agency (FEMA) data, the *Washington Post* discovered that Pence seemed to have moved a decimal point over: Project Airbridge on average had actually delivered about 2.2 million surgical masks a day over the program's span. And when it came to the gold standard in masks—the sought-after N95—the record was even worse: Project Airbridge flights distributed just 768,000 N95 masks, while conventional agency efforts had distributed eighty-five million N95 masks by May.

Project Airbridge was just one of the ways the Trump administration used the pandemic to manifest the ideological wet dream of replacing government agencies with private enterprise, and the altruism of social programs with the market principles inspired by Ayn Rand's Objectivist philosophy of greed.

It was not even clear whether the public was benefitting. For the more than $100 million spent on the flights, the public/private split on the distributed supplies was never clear, with some estimates claiming that it was 80 percent private and only 20 percent public.

Six private mega-companies were granted the right to decide where to deliver the supplies. They were also allowed to charge market rate for those supplies they sold for their own profit. The breakdown was said to be somewhere between 80-20 and 50-50.

The federal government had decided that state public officials should compete in the equivalent of a feudal-themed video game, using the tools they had at hand—battle axes, mead, a bag of magic tricks, and a horse—and fighting each other for ventilators, N95 face masks, and other scarce equipment.

The Project Airbridge enterprise was conducted so far off the books that emergency managers and health officials never knew what they were or were not due to receive—or whom to talk to about it. Officials were tearing their hair out in frustration. Jared Moskowitz, the director of Florida's Division of Emergency Management, told the *Post* in May that he couldn't tell whether Project Airbridge supplies had even been delivered to the state, or why vendors were getting 50 percent of the supplies.

"Do the feds tell them where they want it to go?" he pleaded to journalists. "Or is it the vendor that then gets to decide which order to fill? And how is that even decided? Is it based on how old the order was? Is it based on price? Is it based on need? There's no visibility on any of that."

In April, a group of Democratic senators, led by Elizabeth Warren, opened an investigation into the operation, citing the administration's secrecy. They sent a letter to Cardinal Health, Concordance, Henry Schein, McKesson, Medline, and Owens & Minor, requesting explanations for reports of "political favoritism, cronyism, and price-gouging" in the ongoing supply project. "Taxpayers have shelled out tens of millions of dollars on this secretive project and they deserve to know whether it actually helped get critical supplies to the areas most in need," Warren said in June.

Three of the six suppliers gave the senators copies of memorandums of agreement (MOAs) indicating "that suppliers had complete discretion about how to distribute supplies across hotspot counties" and that "nothing in the MOAs appears to prevent a supplier from sending all of its supplies designated for hotspots to just a single customer in one of the hotspots." The government also hadn't put any kind of conditions on cost: the Justice Department stated that it was none of its business to ask how suppliers arrived at their pricing.

Using taxpayer funds to grease private enrichment was, in fact, a Trump family tradition, going back to the Eisenhower years when Donald Trump's father, Fred, fleeced the government of millions of dollars in loans aimed at housing World War II veterans. Hauled down to Capitol Hill to explain himself, the New York builder was unrepentant, arguing that a loophole in the law allowed for his private gain, and, given that, only a fool would leave all that money on the table. Furthermore, in Trumpworld, only real chumps pay taxes.

That tradition synced up nicely with the goals of the Heritage and Cato foundations, whose minions were quietly leafing through their government-shrinking fantasy football playbooks. The pandemic offered an unprecedented opportunity to go live after decades of tabletop exercises.

As hospital workers pleaded for help, the White House maintained its focus on its conviction that private enterprise was the way out of this disaster. The administration called for volunteers to staff what would become another public/private bonanza, the White House COVID-19 Supply Chain Task Force, helmed by Trump's Mr. Fix-It-All, Jared Kushner.

Kushner had an MBA and hung out with Silicon Valley disruptors, and he was credited with the cheap Facebook ad campaign that got his father-in-law elected in 2016. A group of dewy-eyed, inexperienced young people answered his call, fresh MBAs with nothing in their experience that could have prepared them to understand what they were about to be asked to do—much like Kushner himself. Like so much else in the administration's response, they were off the books—instructed to use their own laptops and personal email accounts, or, better yet, encrypted communication apps like WhatsApp. Eventually, they would be forced to sign the sine qua non of service in Trumpworld, the nondisclosure agreement (NDA).

We don't know what, if anything, this cadre accomplished. At one point, they reportedly had high hopes, an ambitious testing and contact-tracing plan. But according to author Katherine Eban, who first reported on it, the plan was ditched for political reasons. "The political folks believed that because it was going to be relegated to Democratic states, that they could blame those governors, and that would be an effective political strategy," a source told Eban.

The volunteers seem to have been a fresh-faced front office for a more tightly controlled profiteering operation involving networks connected to Kushner and his college roommate, Adam Boehler (overseeing a vast pot of taxpayer money in the Trump administration–created US International Development Finance Corporation), and others in the administration, who could cut deals with private contractors outside normal government channels.

Twenty-six-year-old Max Kennedy Jr., a grandson of Robert F. Kennedy, was one of the volunteers. He joined the task force when the pandemic put his college on hold, and eventually broke his NDA, writing to Congress and talking to journalists and the filmmaker Alex Gibney. He described a surreal supply acquisition and distribution operation handed off to young people without any logistics experience, operating without direction from or interaction with grown-ups from FEMA or anywhere in the government.

"It was the number of people who show up to an after-school event, not to run the greatest crisis in a hundred years," Kennedy said in an interview with Jane Mayer after he resigned. "The fact that they didn't want to get any more people was so upsetting. . . . We were the entire frontline team for the federal government."

Political appointees occasionally dropped in on the group of youngsters, when they needed an assist in the crisis comms operation. One of Trump's political appointees, Brad Smith, tasked Kennedy to create a model that projected the total number of US Covid fatalities at one hundred thousand—a vastly lower number than academics and public health experts had projected. Kennedy, who had no expertise in data modeling, declined.

What looked like chaos from the outside was in fact a deliberate effort to disengage the federal government and leave the blame and logistics problems to the Covid-afflicted states, at the time mostly Democrat-run. Kennedy heard political appointees bragging that Trump "personally came up with the strategy of blaming the states." Other sources credited Kushner, who at some point in his flailing supply chain project calculated that, one, it wasn't going to work and, two, the virus was mainly killing urban people in blue states, a natural selection boon to Trump's election that could be blamed on Democratic officials.

CONTRACT BY TWEET

One thing the shadow operators on the task force did accomplish was creating a list of preferred suppliers. One of them was Yaron Oren-Pines, the Silicon Valley entrepreneur New York State turned to in its hour of darkest desperation with a multi-million-dollar contract.

The Oren-Pines story begins on March 24, when New York governor Andrew Cuomo begged the federal government to help the state get more ventilators for the coming surge of coronavirus patients. At the time, hooking patients up to ventilators was best practice—doctors only later came to understand that the tricky disease could be foiled in advance of that for many patients with anticlotting and steroid medication.

"How can you have New Yorkers possibly dying because they can't get a ventilator?" asked Cuomo. Three days later, President Trump tweeted, "General Motors must . . . start making ventilators, now! Ford, get going on ventilators, fast!"

Oren-Pines, an electrical engineer, tweeted back at him, "We can supply ICU ventilators, invasive and non-invasive." Within days, he turned up on a list vetted by Kushner's team of volunteers, and at their recommendation, officials in New York closed the deal—for $86 million.

The problem was, Oren-Pines had no ventilators and had never been in the medical supply business. He was a classic Silicon Valley macher who had co-founded a networking company: numerous LLCs, properties in San Jose, kids in a Los Gatos private school, Sunnyvale address, married to a photogenic Russian online-chess master with her own IMDb page.

When Oren-Pines failed to deliver, Wells Fargo froze his account and New York canceled the order and demanded the money back. As of this writing, the state is still trying to collect $10 million Oren-Pines is refusing to return.

The Oren-Pines caper wasn't an isolated example. Many more millions of dollars went astray.

Someone inside the government put in a $52 million shipment for Covid tests from the United Arab Emirates. The tests were never picked up, the bill never paid. Months later, HHS informed the seller that it couldn't pay because it couldn't find "any warranted United States contracting officer" involved in the deal.

In May, the director of BARDA, Rick Bright, filed an official whistleblower complaint alleging that Dr. Robert Kadlec, an HHS political appointee and a former Air Force colonel, was participating in multiple schemes to funnel contracts to politically connected companies. Bright was pushed out of the government, even though federal law officially protects whistleblowers.

COVID DEATH RACE

While sharps like Oren-Pines drilled wildcat gushers of cash off the Trump administration's Covid strategy and political appointees like Kadlec steered contracts, President Trump was sneering at governors, telling them to compete with each other for supplies and abide by market principles in which "price is always a component." When asked what states needed to do to get federal help, he smirked that he might help governors who showed him "appreciation."

The first people to understand they were players in this surreal video game, call it *Covid Death Race*, were the governors. On the grim day schools, bars, and restaurants were shutting down across the country, March 16, Trump got on a call with the nation's governors. "We're backing you a hundred percent," he said, before clarifying that he was abdicating leadership and that there was no national plan. "Although respirators, ventilators, all the equipment—try getting it yourselves."

Washington governor Jay Inslee couldn't believe his ears. He said it was as if FDR, the day after Pearl Harbor, had told Connecticut to go build its own battleships.

Governor Cuomo of New York didn't have time to come up with metaphors. New York City was screaming with sirens, bodies were piling up in hospital hallways, and medics and doctors were left without PPE or even a protocol for treating patients. Cuomo was soon reduced to pleading for ventilators on national television, while privately asking why states needed to bid against each other, driving up prices when FEMA could be the sole purchaser.

Adding insult to injury, Kushner proclaimed that Cuomo was overreacting. He was consulting not state or CDC numbers but his own stream of data—provided by Silicon Valley chums running algorithms—and it indicated otherwise.

Now the chaos game was on. The administration would not pool the states into a single buyer, thereby magnifying their ability to bargain down. Rather, Trump continued to tweet personal insults at governors to shame the states into fighting against each other, acting like a "market," and competing.

Incredibly, the feds also started seizing supplies. The governor of Maryland, Republican Larry Hogan, fearing that the federal government would seize a shipment of half a million South Korean Covid tests ordered for his state, instructed the Maryland National Guard to hide them. Hogan told reporters he did this because the feds had seized a shipment of three million N95 masks purchased by Massachusetts at the port of New York. The desperate governor of Rhode Island finally got hold of someone at FEMA who assured her a truckload of federal supplies was on its way. A truck did arrive soon afterward—empty.

Later they would say, as Trump's fourth chief of staff, Mark Meadows, did, that really nothing could be done about the pandemic. All Democrats could do was charge incompetence.

But mostly it was deliberate. The pandemic offered the federal government an opportunity to prove to Americans that government can still be a force for good. Instead, the government did what it could to make sure that whatever remained of that faith after three years of state-smashing ideology would evaporate.

At every decision point, those in the Trump regime chose ideology over compassion, politics over science, opportunism over competence.

Reversing the truth, they politicized the advice of doctors who suggested that mask wearing could hinder transmission of the airborne virus, and turned masks into a signal of totalitarianism.

They stopped the US Postal Service from sending a mask to every address in America.

Trump's surgeon general told Americans not to wear masks.

They threw out the pandemic playbook.

They refused to use two powerful tools, the national stockpile of millions of pieces of PPE and the Defense Production Act.

The act was passed during the height of Cold War, at a time close enough to World War II that the concept of a government order to private enterprise didn't immediately provoke a segment of the citizenry to reach for their guns. But it smelled of socialism. To force industry into production at the behest of some central state office reminded Trump regime donors and diehards of Stalin.

The administration did trigger the law to compel businesses to manufacture equipment, but by midsummer the HHS could only name nineteen companies that were contracted under the act to produce supplies, including six hundred million N95 face masks and respirators. The effort was half-hearted, almost meaningless. Only about half the masks ordered were scheduled for delivery by the end of 2020.

White House trade adviser Peter Navarro claimed that the mere suggestion of the act's powers had been sufficient. "One of the beauties of using the Defense Production Act when necessary is that it has reduced the need to actually have to invoke it because we get voluntary contribution," he said.

Finally, the administration took aim at the pillar of science—the data.

"Everyone wants to describe the day that the light switch flipped and the CDC was sidelined," former CDC chief of staff Kyle McGowan, a Trump political appointee who lost faith in the White House, later recounted to the *New York Times*. "It didn't happen that way. It was more like a hand grasping something, and it slowly closes, closes, closes, closes until you realize, in the middle of the summer, it has a complete grasp on everything at the CDC."

It was hard to pinpoint when exactly the Trump administration destroyed the CDC. Was it when White House officials, on the receiving end of Trump's rage at the stock market crash, told the CDC that the president no longer needed regular telephone briefings with Dr. Messonnier, because he "had his own daily briefings"?

Was it when White House senior adviser Kellyanne Conway weighed in on the rights of churchgoers to gather and sing, or when Ivanka Trump weighed in on schools?

Was it in early summer, when Dr. Redfield capitulated to the White House budget director over changing the CDC's social-distancing guidelines for restaurants so there would be no mention of the six-foot distance?

Was it when the White House started meddling with the CDC's "Morbidity and Mortality Weekly Report," until then the global model for a communicable disease bulletin, devoted to accurate and up-to-date information on infectious diseases? Called the "holiest of the holy" for its scientific inviolability, the report fell victim to Trump political appointees in the health agency who, acting in the interests of the president's 2020 reelection, began pushing to alter or leave out data.

I like the numbers low.

Was it when the Trump administration redirected $250 million from the CDC during the summer to the office of a bullying political hack at the HHS, for a disastrous election year PR campaign to "defeat despair," which went nowhere because celebs didn't want to team up with the Trumpers?

We know how it ends, of course. But we may have forgotten how it unraveled.

"I WANT THEM ALL INFECTED"

Forgive me, gentle reader, for pelting you with a final barrage of WTFs.

As summer rolled on, the Trump election effort took precedence over reducing the death toll. The need for everyone to "be happy" and manipulate numbers grew increasingly frenzied. Messengers of bad numbers were enemies of the political campaign.

Trump himself announced at a Tulsa, Oklahoma, open-air, mask-free campaign rally (his first after the Covid lockdown started in March) that he had ordered his staff to "slow the testing down."

That rally turned out to be a superspreader event, resulting in a Covid surge in Oklahoma and the death of Herman Cain, a Trump supporter and former GOP presidential candidate. It also was so sparsely attended that Trump flew into a rage and later demoted his campaign manager, Brad Parscale, who would shortly attain a second round of notoriety by getting arrested in his underwear outside his Florida manse for pulling a gun on his wife.

Meanwhile, hacks at the HHS were seething with paranoia. They accused CDC scientists of cooking data and science to try to kill Trump's reelection chances.

In one late-summer email, an HHS science adviser named Paul Alexander wrote: "CDC tried to report as if once kids get together, there will be spread and this will impact school reopening. . . . Very misleading by CDC and shame on them. Their aim is clear. . . . This is designed to hurt this Presidnet [*sic*] for their reasons which I am not interested in." Alexander had advocated for herd immunity while the HHS officially denied it supported that goal. "We want them infected," he advised, of infants, children, and teens. He criticized the CDC for pointing out that the virus was disproportionately killing minorities, arguing that their deaths were due to "decades of democrat [*sic*] neglect."

Dr. Redfield tried to delete Alexander's missives before congressional investigators got hold of them.

Alexander's protégé at the HHS was a political operator who graduated from the Roger Stone School of Ratfuck named Michael Caputo. Caputo's job was communications. But as the facts increasingly were at odds with the Trump reelection campaign's PR needs, Caputo fell apart, announcing on Facebook that people needed to stock up on ammunition, because "deep state scientists" were plotting "sedition" together at coffee shops. After the *New York Times* reported on the outburst, Caputo took a sixty-day "medical leave." He and Alexander both left the government shortly thereafter.

Americans wouldn't wear masks and wouldn't stay home. No leader stood before them at the beginning, explained what was happening, and asked for their cooperation and sacrifice.

No leader had made such an ask of Americans for a long time, not since World War II, really.

Certainly, Trump would not be that man.

Not now, not with 40 percent of the population obese and so unhealthy that only about half of applicants can even pass the health requirements to enter the all-volunteer military.

The virus would feast on Americans. There was no medicine to save those who got sickest, the one in five hospitalized. They would be dying by the hundreds of thousands before the end of the year.

The only hope was a vaccine.

CHAPTER 2

Vaccine

*People have been living on earth for about
250,000 years. For the past 5,000 years, healers have been
trying to heal the sick. For all but the past 200,
they haven't been very good at it.*

—DR. PAUL OFFIT, from *Do You Believe in Magic?*

What doesn't kill me makes me stronger.

—FRIEDRICH NIETZSCHE

The fur-clad roamers of the steppe who left no monuments gave us the word in their Proto-Indo-European language: *wokeha*. Over millennia, it evolved, but it is still recognizable. *Vaca* in ancient Rome and Spain today. *Baqara* in Arabic. *Vache* in French.

Cow. Giver of milk and cream, cheese, yogurt, T-bones and hamburgers, cow pies—and vaccine.

It is right that our word for a life-saving inoculation is related to an ancient word for "cow." Humankind is microbially intertwined with the bovine. Over tens of thousands of years that we have lived in proximity with ruminants and other domesticated and some wild beasts, their microbes became ours. Like the bat-nestled coronavirus that has, we are told, morphed from remote cave dweller to pandemic Covid, many of man's deadliest bacteria and viruses are related to other animal diseases that naturally evolved to sicken or kill us. (Bacteria are the larger of the two microorganisms; viruses, besides being smaller, require living hosts to multiply.)

Measles. Plague. Tuberculosis. Smallpox. The big four all have analogues in the animals that we have kept, or attracted with our food and filth. So do many others.

For millennia, humanity had one weapon against all epidemics—luck. Plague, cholera, typhoid arrived, sickened some and killed others without rhyme or reason, and then disappeared. In retrospect, the seers and wise ones could always look back on the signs—a comet or some other astrological conjunction, a tribal victory to be avenged, failures to sufficiently supplicate the gods. Infectious disease, waves of contagion, wiped out pauper, king, everyone in between and sometimes whole civilizations. People could only fall to their knees and pray to a great supernatural being to protect themselves and their loved ones.

The role of disease in shaping world history, and man's feeble attempts to evade, suppress, control, and conquer epidemics, is a story that will be written and rewritten as long as human beings walk the face of the earth.

But modern medicine—arriving in the late 1700s, the beginning of our era in terms of scientific method—gave our species its first real fighting chance. From the lowly cowpox vaccine (more on that below), to advances in lens grinding that enabled humans to see previously invisible killers, to the age of experiments (conducted long before electricity or indoor plumbing or, certainly, supercomputers) that revealed which bugs did what to us and what we could do to kill or control them—all that happened in the last three hundred years, with the most significant scientific discoveries occurring in just the last 150 years. This leap in understanding is so vast and so much part of our modern world that we tend to take it for granted.

Before the birth of early modern science in the eighteenth century, human beings were helpless against all infectious disease. Plague, carried by fleas on rats, ravaged Europe and Asia over recorded history, wiping out whole cities and altering the course of civilization. The Old Testament speaks of plagues as one of a just and unforgiving God's punishments. Pagan Lucretius recorded the grisly details of the plague of Athens in 430 BCE that emerged from "deep within Egypt's bounds." According to that account, the plague started with a fever and a headache, then covered the throat in ulcers so that "blood trickles from the tongue," and then flowed into the lungs and heart. The fevers and unquenchable thirst were so tormenting that, the writer claimed, the dying flung themselves into rivers and wells and drowned.

The Black Death, centuries later, carried off a nearly civilization-ending 50 percent of Europe. In the long, dark years before microbiology proved the germ theory of illness, even the best doctors and philosophers had no idea what caused disease. Proto-doctors advised people to avoid fogs, swamps, miasmas, and places that smelled bad, and to mind the astrologers, but beyond that they were ignorant of the cause, utterly blind to the microbial world. When plague struck, people carried pockets full of posies to protect themselves from the disease-causing bad smells.

The rich, as today, could flee cities when sickness came, and often survived by isolating themselves. Well into the eighteenth century, the doors of the epidemic-stricken in European cities were nailed shut and scrawled with a "plague cross" in red.

Those left behind in population centers could only cordon off the sick and seek quack prophylactics, like the Londoners who pinned dead toads to their collars to ward off plague in Daniel Defoe's account of a seventeenth-century outbreak.

Epidemics surged and waned, carried across continents by caravans on trade routes or across waters by ships port to port, or armies marching on long journeys, as the world grew more interconnected. So the arrival of plague was always understood to have come from "somewhere else." One nation blamed another; it came from Italy or Egypt, always carried by strangers. The Italian *quarantina*, meaning "forty"—referring to the forty days ships were held at port before passengers, who were feared to carry the plague, could disembark—gave us the word "quarantine," now connected with air travel. One can find remnants of quarantine sectors, sometimes converted to parks and often containing a mossy cemetery, in almost every European port city.

SMALLPOX

Of the great epidemics of history, smallpox was among the most terrible. It inflicted gruesome torment, killing hundreds of millions and sometimes wiping out whole peoples, like many indigenous American populations. Weeping sores covered every inch of skin, and victims remained conscious as their flesh disintegrated. Survivors were disfigured for life, physically and emotionally.

Smallpox had a milder analogue in a cow pathogen called cowpox, a mild rash that didn't kill animals or humans. Weeping sores that resembled the ones produced by smallpox appeared on the udders of milking cows and did sometimes infect the hands of milkmaids and farmhands—but without killing them.

According to medical legend, in the late 1700s an English country doctor named Edward Jenner encountered a milkmaid who claimed to be immune to smallpox because she had already suffered from the related disease that afflicted cows' udders. As the legend goes, Jenner took a bit of the milkmaid's cowpox scab and scratched the pus into the skin of a boy named James Phipps, who then proved immune to smallpox, along with other children Jenner experimented on, including his own eleven-month-old son.

Jenner's vaccine was in fact a cure that had been known for a long time already in Asia. As early as the fifteenth century CE, the Chinese understood that people who had smallpox and didn't die of it never got it again. They began applying small amounts of dried smallpox scab to healthy people to protect them from full-blown disease.

The practice was already widespread in the Ottoman lands by the time Lady Mary Wortley Montagu traveled to Constantinople in 1716 with her diplomat husband. Lady Mary's brother had died of smallpox, and she herself had survived it but with her face forever scarred. On her travels around the Ottoman Empire, she learned of a practice that was believed to prevent smallpox. Healer women who stored scrapings of smallpox scabs in nutshells visited families in their homes. The healer would ask each where they wanted to be inoculated, make a small incision, then take a bit of the pox substance and rub it into a vein or cut.

The British soon adopted this practice, with doctors going door to door administering the inoculation. It usually worked, but sometimes it provoked the real disease and killed the patient. They knew, without perhaps verbalizing it or under-standing why, that what didn't kill them made them stronger.

Enter the cow.

The origin of the *variolae vaccinae*—Latin for the "smallpox of the cow"—begins with a doctor named John Fewster, who learned of the cowpox and farmhands' immunity to smallpox in 1768 while infecting them with tiny bits of smallpox in the Asian style. The practice was risky—it killed one out of every fifty people—but many submitted because it was better odds than the one in six who died after catching it naturally.

Fewster shared his observations about the farmhands and the cowpox at the eighteenth-century version of a medical con-ference—over bottles of port or brandy with fellow medical men at a local inn called the Ship. Edward Jenner, then a young apprentice, heard Fewster's story and became so obsessed that his friends at the inn nicknamed him "the Cowpox Bore."

Thirty years later, after his own career as a country doctor brought him into repeated contact with the cowpox-immunity phenomenon, Jenner first vaccinated that small boy with a milk-maid's cowpox—earning sole credit for the idea, and putting the milkmaid at the center of the legend.

STEAMPUNK SCIENCE

In the eighteenth century, life was still, by our standards, nasty, brutish, and short. But science was inching into modernity. Researchers were moving beyond alchemy and astrology and priests and the quasi-supernatural medicine of the ancients. The Hippocratic four "humors" (choleric, sanguine, phleg-matic, and melancholic) and their related bodily fluids (yellow bile, blood, phlegm, and black bile) would remain a factor in medical science for another century. But deductive reasoning, classification and experimentation, and systematic hypothesis testing all brought new ideas and new technologies, especially the microscope. With eyes on the microbial world for the first time, researchers came to a new understanding of infectious disease.

In the years immediately following Jenner's invention, the vaccine was only applied against smallpox. A host of other infectious diseases, bacterial and viral, continued to kill adults and children or shorten lives, or at the very least make them miserable. But not even the most modern doctors of the eighteenth and early nineteenth centuries would have believed that tiny creatures—and not miasmas or bad air or individual constitutions—determined who got sick and when and how.

Then a new breed of researcher appeared on the scene. The early nineteenth-century microbe hunters were the first to try to understand bacteria and viruses and their roles in sickness. The names of many of the early microbe hunters are mostly forgotten, other than that of the great Louis Pasteur.

They made discoveries using the rudimentary lenses available in that pre-electrified era. Inside their gaslit laboratories, experimenters with steampunk technology began to make out the blurry outlines of the once invisible enemy.

Even after they saw the "beasties" or "animalcules," it took many more years to suss out the ones that killed. First, they saw the spores of anthrax, then the tiny rods of tuberculosis, then the comma-shaped killers inside the guts of cholera victims. The new understanding took some decades to prevail. As late as the 1880s, the old bulls of science in Europe resisted the notion that these invisible creatures had murdered millions of human beings. It was hard to let go of the age-old notion that the spiritual/biological ephemera of individual "constitutions" caused sickness—especially when deadly germs sometimes left people unaffected, like when the old German professor, to the horror of his younger colleagues, once drank a vial of live cholera bacteria to disprove the theory. "Germs are of no account in cholera!" Professor Max Josef von Pettenkofer of Munich supposedly shouted after surviving the cholera cocktail, according to microbe-hunter historian Paul de Kruif. "The important thing is the *disposition* of the individual."

Sorting out which viruses sickened humans was a great challenge in those early years. Viruses are the most common active particles on earth. A mind-bending number of them—10 to the 31st power—populate the planet. The early researchers' task was made even more difficult by the fact that viruses are not even "alive" outside cells. They are inert and can only reproduce inside other plant or animal life.

Vaccines against viruses besides smallpox began to proliferate after these early researchers learned how to grow viruses in serum or eggs or lab animals. Once they could tell what was killing people, they could try to weaken the viruses, in the manner of the naturally weaker cowpox, and make protective vaccines. Many first tested the resulting vaccine fluid on themselves or their own children. Eventually, lab animals replaced that practice. Countless mice and monkeys, dogs, guinea pigs, and other mammals would be—and mice still are today—martyred to the cause of extending human life.

The French chemist and microbiologist Pasteur, whose name is commemorated in processes to keep wine and milk bacteria-free, is the best known but not the only great genius of nineteenth-century microbial research. He produced the world's second vaccine, against rabies, testing it on a boy savagely bitten by a rabid dog. Pasteur's vaccine worked on the same principle as Jenner's cowpox/smallpox model. He injected attenuated rabies vaccine into the injured boy, who not only survived but lived to a ripe old age working as a gatekeeper for the Pasteur Institute in Paris, dying in 1940. The Pasteur Institute went on to produce the first lab-created vaccine in 1879, against chicken cholera, and attracted scientists from around Europe, and it is still advancing biological sciences today.

It took another fifty years for science to design the next major human vaccine, against yellow fever. Yellow fever epidemics were common in the warmer regions of the globe, including parts of the United States. For centuries (it was first identified in the 1500s, probably as Europeans began to travel to the tropics), the transmission of yellow fever was an utter mystery. The virus attacked the liver, producing jaundice, hence the name. Yellow fever wiped out 10 percent of the population of Philadelphia in the early 1800s, a disaster that doctors like Benjamin Rush, signer of the Declaration of Independence, could do nothing about. Victims received palliative care. If they survived, they were immune for life.

In 1900, US Army surgeon Walter Reed (after whom the Bethesda, Maryland, hospital that serves US presidents and veterans of our wars is named) proved that the *Aedes aegypti* mosquito was the carrier of yellow fever. Max Theiler and Hugh Smith grew the virus in eggs, and then passed it from egg to egg. After two hundred eggs, the virus was attenuated and no longer caused disease. Theiler and Smith inoculated half a million Brazilians with this egg-grown virus, effectively ending the scourge in that country in the late 1930s. Unfortunately, this success story came with a disaster. The vaccine used human serum as a base, and 330,000 US soldiers were infected with hepatitis B between

1941 and 1942 because a batch was made with infected blood. Fifty thousand soldiers developed hepatitis.

POLIO

The world's fourth great vaccine was aimed at polio. An American success story, it also marked the beginning of the era of mass immunization and the dawn of the age of vaccine litigation.

Into the mid-twentieth century, the polio virus was a terrifying, tricky microbe. It had afflicted people since antiquity, and is probably depicted on an ancient Egyptian statue of a stooped and crippled man. But polio was relatively rare until the 1800s, when the disease surged for reasons that may have to do with a paradox of modern sanitation. One theory is that cleaner cities and towns prevented babies from coming into contact with the polio virus while still covered by maternal immunity. When they encountered it later as children or adults, maternal immunity had worn off, and they got sick.

Polio stalked in waves. It crept up on communities in spring and peaked in August or September, making summer breaks a time of terror for parents whose children wanted to frolic at parks and on beaches and in swimming pools. Polio thrived in densely packed cities like New York. Epidemics in 1894 and 1916 crippled thousands and challenged the metropolitan public health authorities. Panicked residents did exactly what citizens of ancient Rome or medieval Genoa and London did when the plague struck. They turned to quack and natural cures: eating catnip, skullcap, lady's slipper, earthworm oil, blackberry brandy, even the blood of frogs, snakes, and horses, and hanging charms around their necks of pepper, garlic, camphor, and onions.

The polio virus lives in the intestine, an enterovirus that reproduces in the gut and is transmitted by feces and contaminated water. It only sickens a small percentage of its carriers. Less than 1 percent of victims develop paralytic polio, in which the virus leaves the digestive tract, enters the bloodstream, and then attacks spinal nerve cells. In severe cases, it paralyzes the throat and chest and, in those cases, victims die without artificial breathing support.

As with so many other epidemic diseases, doctors could only offer general advice on how to avoid exposure and provide palliative care. During the spring and summer season, doctors and families were on high alert for the early signs—a headache, vomiting, neck stiffness—followed by the terrible paralysis in the limbs and eventually in the lungs.

Fifteen thousand Americans were paralyzed annually in the 1950s.

For those whose lungs were affected, the iron lung was the last resort. Doctors placed the supine victim into a metal tube, so that only his or her head protruded, while the mechanical device used air pressure to force air into and out of the patient's lungs, in hopes that the patient would recover enough to eventually breathe unaided. Fully paralyzed women were even known to give birth in the iron lung. Some remained in the iron lung for a year or more. Survival rates often depended on age—better for younger sufferers—with some destined to live out their lives in the machines.

Meanwhile, modern science could now be applied to vaccine research. Much had changed since the development of the smallpox vaccine nearly two hundred years prior. Scientists now understood the role of microbes in illness—polio was first identified in 1908. Pasteur's scientific descendants were specializing in new and specific areas of germ study, including virology. Less depended on chance, more on scientific method and experience. Researchers now had a variety of options for growing and measuring viruses, and basic technology enabling more precise targeting of infectious pathogens.

The first American polio vaccine was developed in the wake of the New York epidemics by a Temple University doctor, John Kolmer, who had developed a blood test for syphilis and famously had tried and failed to save President Calvin Coolidge's teenage son from staph infection. Kolmer developed his vaccine by infecting monkeys with polio, taking their polio-ravaged spines and crushing them, and then killing the live virus in a solution of ricin—the deadly substance extracted from the castor bean that is now better known as a bioweapon.

Kolmer tested the resulting vaccine first on his own sons, ages eleven and fifteen, and an assistant and then twenty-five other children, all of whom survived. In 1934, he received approval to make enough to vaccinate ten thousand children. Since it took one monkey spine to make forty doses, tens of thousands of monkeys were killed for human health.

At the same time, another doctor, Maurice Brodie of New York University, was experimenting with polio-infected monkey spinal cord material attenuated in formaldehyde. He injected himself and five coworkers and then got the green light to test it more widely.

The test subjects for the two vaccines, however, were not as lucky as the two doctors and their family members and assistants. The trick with attenuated pathogen vaccines is to find the right balance. Too strong, and the vaccinated catch the disease. Too weak, and it has no protective effect. Sufficient amounts of live virus apparently eluded the ricin and formaldehyde and made it into the vaccine vials, and into the arms of young people. The vaccines paralyzed ten children and killed at least five. Although polio was to remain one of the nation's leading epidemic diseases, these disastrous accidents put a stop to polio vaccine testing for another two decades.

The search for a cure gained support again in the 1940s. In August 1921, future president Franklin Delano Roosevelt was thirty-nine, a hale and hearty American aristocrat who sailed, rode horseback, and lived like one of the charmed characters out of an F. Scott Fitzgerald story. On his annual summer vacation at the Roosevelt family compound on an island off the coast of Maine, he woke up with a headache and lost feeling in his legs soon after. FDR was diagnosed with polio, spent the rest of his life paralyzed from the waist down, and never gave up searching for a cure.

FDR's celebrity launched national fund-raisers like the March of Dimes (millions of Americans mailed in a dime or two) and raised millions of dollars. In 1938, the money helped finance a new organization, the National Foundation for Infantile Paralysis (NFIP), which would in turn devote money and expertise to new research for a vaccine.

The NFIP granted its first $200,000 to a star virologist, Jonas Salk. With a large staff of fifty and an even larger lab of monkeys, Salk resurrected the vaccine made of polio virus— this time bred in monkey kidney cells—and inactivated by formaldehyde. In 1952, when polio surged and fifty-eight thousand Americans were sickened, Salk sped up his work. In 1953, the NFIP organized Salk's first large-scale trial, vaccinating four hundred thousand children—successfully.

Salk then shared his technique with pharmaceutical companies, with the aim of a much larger vaccination campaign.

In the spring of 1954, the national public health authorities launched the greatest mass vaccination effort in the nation's history, aiming to ultimately vaccinate millions of children.

What happened next changed the course of vaccine research and production, and left traces of vaccine distrust in the general culture that have never disappeared. Salk's method of inactivating the virus in formaldehyde worked on small batches. But at industrial scale, it turned out that the live virus managed to survive the process. The problem existed at all large production efforts, but the bigger companies had fail-safes that prevented them from delivering contaminated doses into arms.

One small family-owned California lab, Cutter (known today among campers for its bug spray), however, did not have those fail-safes in place. Cutter had made its name in veterinary medicine for more than a century. Its lab produced the vaccine according to Salk's instructions. But live polio virus made it through the formaldehyde and the company's glass filters.

Within weeks of a 1955 polio vaccination round involving two hundred thousand children in western and midwestern states, children who had received the Cutter vaccine started showing up sick. Some were paralyzed within days. Eventually, the US government shut down the polio vaccination effort.

An investigation confirmed the problems and the main source of the contaminated virus. Men in the chain of command in the US public health apparatus were fired. But the larger companies went back to the labs and proved that they could filter their product successfully.

Another polio outbreak in 1955 provoked the government to resume mass polio vaccinations. To get teens to cooperate, Elvis Presley even joined the cause and submitted to a vaccination photo op backstage before an appearance on *The Ed Sullivan Show* in 1956.

By the 1960s and 1970s, polio was on the way to being vanquished in America, as childhood vaccinations became not only routine but required. But the damage was done. The widely publicized polio vaccination incidents left a seed of distrust that sprouted and blossomed over the years, and confounds public health officials to this day.

Today, some American parents balk at having their squirming child be injected with a supposedly lifesaving serum if there is even a slim chance the serum could kill or paralyze their child.

The contaminated polio vaccines spawned precedent-setting lawsuits that forever changed the way US companies designed and put products on the market—especially medical products. The first lawsuit against Cutter was brought by the family of a California child, paralyzed for life at age eight by the vaccine. Their attorney, the showboating plaintiff lawyer Melvin Belli (who would go on to represent the Rolling Stones, Muhammad Ali, and Zsa Zsa Gabor, among a number of other celebrities), persuaded a small-town California jury that even if they didn't believe Cutter was negligent, they could and should find Cutter liable for the damage its product had done.

"It is going to change the face of the legal map," a gleeful Belli said at the time.

The verdict putting the onus on corporations without requiring proof of negligence opened the door to countless other product liability lawsuits. And it chilled pharmaceutical innovation for years to come—but especially with respect to vaccines, which are typically low-profit and administered on a mass scale, increasing the risk of an adverse event.

After the Cutter debacle, pharmaceutical companies would

shy away from researching vaccines—away from any new inventions that might have a broad public health effect but would bring in very little financial return, and potentially costly lawsuits.

For about sixty years, until Covid, the number of companies producing vaccines dwindled. In 2019, only five companies were still making vaccines for use in the United States.

Jonas Salk was a controversial man of science—loathed by colleagues for his ego and unwillingness to share credit, but a celebrity in American popular culture. In 1968, the United States replaced his vaccine with an oral version, supposedly safer, designed by the Russian virologist Albert Sabin. Sabin attenuated his live virus by reproducing it hundreds of times in monkey cells. Children gobbled up the weakened virus on sugar cubes into the 1990s—despite the fact that even it delivered traces of dangerous virus on occasion and caused some paralysis over the years.

Today, Salk's vaccine is the one US children start to get at just two months of age.

THE FLU SHOT

Besides routine childhood immunizations, the vaccine most Americans are most familiar with is the flu shot. Hippocrates first described what was probably flu in the fourth century BCE, and flu viruses and epidemics have occurred around the world throughout recorded history. The name "influenza" was coined in sixteenth-century Italy by a writer who attributed a pandemic that affected Europe, Africa, and Asia to the "influence" of the stars.

The last great global pandemic was the 1918–19 Spanish flu, a terrifying and deadly disease that infected a third of the world's population and killed upward of fifty million people—though fewer than one million in the United States—in waves of death around the globe. The virus felled young and healthy adults, sometimes within twenty-four hours, attacking their lungs so that they filled with fluid and literally drowned them in their own immune response. The pandemic only ended after enough people had been sick that doctors could start injecting people with antibodies made from convalescent plasma.

During the Spanish flu epidemic, scientists still believed the flu was bacterial, but the epidemic prompted a round of research and development, so that by the 1930s, researchers discovered the influenza A virus, and further strains B and C, which were less virulent than A. In 1938, the first inactivated live virus vaccine was authorized for military use. Among the doctors who worked on it was Jonas Salk, who would apply flu virus vaccine research to his future work with polio.

Throughout history, soldiers had always died more often from disease than they did on the battlefield, but during the 1918–19 outbreak, flu accounted for roughly half of US military casualties in Europe. It arguably led to the end of World War I.

Two decades later, as the United States geared up for World War II, war planners were keenly aware of how the flu had ravaged troops in Europe, and in 1941 the US Army organized a commission to develop the first flu vaccine, dragooning top specialists from universities, hospitals, public health labs, and private foundations into the effort. The all-hands federal effort broke new ground in vaccine technology generally. It also led to a separate line of research, potentially much more sinister: the search for biological weapons—an effort that would feed a vast distrust of science and the rise of worldwide conspiracy

theories around the weaponizing of medical research and vaccines. I'll be addressing this in chapter 4.

Refinements to flu virus vaccines continued throughout the
twentieth century, as mutated flu viruses caused new pandemics
(the 1968 Hong Kong flu was especially deadly), requiring new
waves of research and new vaccines. Since these outbreaks were
global, the WHO started flu-monitoring projects in the 1960s.
And researchers by the 1990s had applied new technology,
including recombinant DNA, to speed production of vaccines
that had to be altered for every new flu virus.

AIDS

For all the vaccine success stories, many diseases still defy
vaccine prophylactics. HIV/AIDS preoccupied a generation
of vaccine researchers. The epidemic, as we know, forged the
careers of all the top public health officials in the initial US
Covid response—Dr. Birx, Dr. Redfield, and Dr. Fauci all cut
their teeth on the government fight against the AIDS virus.

The search for an AIDS vaccine never found its Holy Grail,
but it drove research into new territory, including immunology,
virology, and nucleic acid therapeutics—all of which made
the Covid vaccine possible. In 2019, before Covid landed, Dr.
Fauci cowrote a paper hailing "the collateral advantages of"
HIV studies in advancing new cures and treatments for other
diseases.

AIDS research also raised false hopes. In 1992, Dr. Redfield,
then a colonel based at Walter Reed, got behind an AIDS
vaccine called VaxSyn, claiming it was proven to protect the
immune systems of infected soldiers. The vaccine never worked,
as the AIDS virus is too mutable, but Dr. Redfield talked Con-

gress into financing a $20 million clinical trial on HIV-positive men. After the VaxSyn failure, the US Army investigated Dr. Redfield over his support for it.

The worldwide fight against AIDS coalesced around philanthropies and foundations that played a major role in fighting other diseases on a global scale. Thanks largely to them, global vaccination rates reached all-time highs in the past two decades. For example, in 1999 the Bill & Melinda Gates Foundation announced it would spend $100 million for vaccine research. The Gates Foundation would go on to spend billions vaccinating children in the developing world. Working with other philanthropies and wealthy nations, the Gates Foundation financed research into malaria vaccines and pushed many other vaccines—like the lifesaving anti-diarrhea rotavirus shot—into impoverished African nations.

The efforts paid off: as of 2017, the Gates Foundation was credited with saving 122 million lives. But they also spawned conspiracy theories about Westerners secretly seeding disease among Muslims, or sterilizing children. Some leaders have argued that Gates's wealth would be better spent on social and economic programs that uplift whole societies. Gates's unrivaled power at the forefront of the global vaccine movement sometimes put him in conflict with NGOs with competing interests. It also made him a handy poster boy villain in Covid vaccine conspiracy theories at home.

Until the twentieth century, very few people survived childhood without suffering from the agonies inflicted by infectious diseases themselves, or witnessing family members that did. People died at home. Their survivors—our great-grandparents—were intimately acquainted with the sights and smells and sounds of the stages of death, experiences relegated for the most part now to nurses and hospice workers. Death and disease lay much closer to them than they do to us today.

Viewed from above, vaccines are a massive success story. They have been helping us live longer and safer to a degree unimaginable little more than a century ago. In 1900, the US life expectancy was forty-six for men and forty-eight for women. Someone born in 2019 can expect to live to between seventy-five and eighty years old, although due to health inequities, lifespans vary depending on race, ethnicity, and gender.

The scale of change has been dramatic. But it can be hard to see. We belong to the most medically protected generation in human history, and that protection has made us both complacent and risk-averse.

The history of twentieth-century vaccine developments is a seesaw between advancements in medical science and conspiracy theories and distrust engendered by its accidents or failures. Almost every new vaccine is accompanied by reports of risk, side effects, and sometimes terrible accidents, at least one involving tens of thousands of sickened people.

Despite the missteps, and legions of paralyzed monkeys and dead mice, vaccines have mostly done their job of eradicating the diseases that once plagued inhabitants of the Global North. The Western Hemisphere was declared polio-free in 1994. Polio still surges occasionally in some African and Asian countries.

The polio vaccine is now one of a regimen of at least fifteen childhood vaccinations that the United States recommends and that children must receive to enter most public schools. Children are now jabbed with serums that create antibodies to hepatitis B, measles, mumps, rubella, diphtheria, tetanus, pertussis—all diseases that well into the twentieth century had spread through communities, killing babies or permanently damaging health.

Vaccines, writes Heidi Larson, founder and director of the London-based Vaccine Confidence Project, represent "one of the biggest worldwide social experiments in collectivism and cooperation in modern times." Larson founded the project in 2010 because in many nations, childhood vaccines have elicited a mass anti-vaccination movement.

Modern mass vaccine efforts always must contend with conspiracy theories and community distrust—of the West, of science, of medicine, or all three. Working around and tamping down conspiracies and distrust is a full-time job for a whole subset of social and medical workers.

THE *WALL-E* GENERATION

The pandemic landed on us at a time when the for-profit American health care system was in many ways inferior to many publicly funded systems in Europe and in many Asian nations. Forty percent of Americans are obese, many with underlying health conditions related to obesity, and the US infant mortality rate ranks higher than that of our peers in the industrial world. About half of new recruits fail the US Army's entry-level physical fitness test. And for probably the first time ever, after steadily increasing for most of our nation's history, the life expectancy of Americans has actually been declining in recent years. All that's before Covid.

Covid emerged from the bat cave at a time when most people in America were vaccinated. In the American mind, epidemics were a thing of the past—or if not the past, they were terrible things that happened very, very far away.

The American medical system still had an international reputation. The sheen of the CDC remained, even if the CDC itself was suddenly on the skids due to political manipulation. American advanced research reigned supreme. The nation boasted some of the best—and highest-paid—private doctors and surgeons and specialists on the planet, albeit available mostly only to the very rich.

Covid would kill hundreds of thousands of Americans, and expose national shortcomings for all the world to see. Even Dr. Redfield, in December 2020 (and perhaps partly to cover over the failings at the CDC under his watch), claimed that the American Covid mortality rate was directly related to the high national obesity rate.

But in January 2020, as Covid was leaking out of China, onto airplanes and cruise ships and into Seattle and New York City, American complacency was such that if you asked the average American on the street, most believed that the United States, with the best doctors and health care in the world, would elude the pandemic.

The false sense of security extended to the experts as well. Virologists and public health planners had been behind several "boy who cried wolf" pandemic scares in the preceding decades. SARS and MERS were killers, but they hadn't jumped the ocean and spread like wildfire. The swine flu was contagious as hell, but it wasn't the killer we'd been warned about. We'd been lucky. The plagues wished on us by our enemies in recent years had not come to pass—not yet.

"There were a lot of fire alarms with no fire, so people tended to ignore this one," Lawrence Gostin, director of Georgetown's O'Neill Institute for National and Global Health Law, told Kaiser Health News to explain why he underestimated the virus in its first few weeks.

The misplaced complacency and out-of-date assumptions about American superiority coincided with a growing antipathy among a sector of Americans toward science and experts. Free marketeers and their handmaidens in politics had been denigrating government and manipulating science and medicine to maximize profits for decade—most famously in the sugar industry's fight with science over obesity, the tobacco/lung cancer "debate," and now the climate change denial movement. This propaganda game had been underway for decades, but Trump's election in 2016 signaled that distrust in experts was now a dominant cultural phenomenon. MAGA essentially upholds the notion that if it was good enough for gramps, it's good enough for me. It promotes "common sense" and DIY investigations and replaces respect for PhDs with resentment toward those who have them and the elitism they represent.

Covid struck America at a perilous moment politically, but also in terms of American hardiness. Modern medicine, including the fifteen vaccines babies in the United States are either required or recommended to receive, had all but erased the infectious diseases that plagued the American people well into the twentieth century. Heart disease and cancer were still killers, but advances in surgery and chemotherapies help improve the odds of survival for patients even against those maladies.

The new disease challenged experts and scientists all over the world at once. Months before Covid made landfall in America, an international body ranking countries' preparedness for a pandemic put the United States at number one. The virus would claim that reputation along with well over half a million American lives.

But the successes of medical science, and especially vaccines, have spoiled us. A significant segment of the generation of men and women who were the greatest beneficiaries of scientific advances in human history had come to distrust, and even scorn and reject, the fruits and methods of science.

Meanwhile, many Americans, especially the poor, are very sick in new and different ways.

The abundance and conveniences of life in the richest nation in the world have sparked a different sort of pandemic. Forty percent of Americans are obese, and significant numbers suffer from obesity's relatives, diabetes and hypertension. And they aren't just old people. A majority of young Americans are also sick with the effects of sloth and abundance and have been for some time.

Covid, it turned out, loved those *WALL-E*-style comorbidities. Loved them to death.

When Covid first swept through New York in the horrible March and April months of 2020, frontline doctors and medics stashed blue-faced gasping people in hospital hallways. New York governor Cuomo put out a call for nurses from the rest of the nation to help attach patients to ventilators and hope for the best. Tens of thousands died anyway. When people's legs turned black, doctors amputated them—until they understood that the disease has a clotting effect that can be mitigated with a small dose of an existing medicine. Surgeons in New York City are traumatized by the memory of hundreds of what turned out to be possibly needless amputations. As the bodies piled up, they learned a little more from each tragic mistake. Still, the disease was wily. Even when their lives were saved, after discharge, weeks or months later, some long-haul survivors had enduring physical and neurological problems, including fatigue, post-Covid brain fog, mental illness, even episodes of psychosis.

By the time the zombie plague began to ravage the entire country, half the population was already habituated to looking at people with training and credentials and sneering, "You think you're pretty smart, doncha?"

The great irony of this, the cosmic joke, is that in the middle of this virulently anti-science era, big brains are riding to the rescue. A new vaccine technology has been perched on the divide between theoretical and practical for decades. The pandemic has provided an opportunity to produce and test—massively and rapidly—a type of nucleotide vaccine platform that has been on the brink of approval and distribution for years.

MOLECULAR MOONSHOTS

All successful vaccines have been improvements on the two-century-old invention of a country doctor working blind in the era before the microscope. Even after the invention of the microscope and later leaps in medical technology, the platform was the same: attenuate or weaken the virus so it cannot reproduce, and inject it into the bloodstreams of the healthy, provoking an immune response to resist the potent virus if and when the immune system encounters it.

Before anyone could "see" the microbial world, we understood that for infectious diseases, what doesn't kill you makes you stronger.

The system worked well but it was never infallible. People suffered from bad side effects; some died. Deadly pathogens, accidents, contamination, too much, too little. Vaccine production is not nimble: it takes time to grow weakened virus in eggs or other fermenters. When swine flu (HINI) jumped from pigs to humans and infected millions, scientists had the means to rapidly identify the virus. But they couldn't cook up a fast vaccine because attenuating the virus in eggs took months. The swine flu vaccine was not released early enough to prevent the first wave of the pandemic, and two hundred thousand people died worldwide.

The Covid pandemic demanded speed.

Almost since Covid entered our consciousness, we've heard the phrase "spike protein" almost as often as "lockdown" and "mask." The spike protein is said to be the virus's special weapon. Television and newspaper imagery has burned the image into our brains—the enemy is a round, spiked ball.

The fact that scientists could even talk about the spike protein indicates how far microbiology has come since the milk-maid and the cowpox. Researchers, aided by supercomputers, advanced chemistry, and other new imaging technologies like X-ray crystallography and cryo-electron microscopy, have assembled a vast war chest of knowledge about the tiniest building blocks of life, and even know how to manipulate and create new viral forms.

For most Americans, the language in that war chest might as well be ancient Greek. The Covid vaccine we are being asked to accept is the product of a new language of medical knowledge and technology. And so it is with the spike protein.

Besides being the sole food allowed on the keto diet, the bar in the hiker's backpack, what is a *protein* anyway?

To biologists, life is chemistry. Proteins are chemicals that control the body's chemical reactions at the cellular level. They are microscopic and myriad and they play a special role in maintaining life. They are like steelworkers in a blast furnace. Proteins "coax and control" basic chemical reactions, "speeding some and slowing others, pacing the reactions just enough to be compatible with living," writes Dr. Siddhartha Mukherjee in his book

The Gene. Dr. Mukherjee describes the incredible specificity and delicacy of their function: "Organisms exist not because of reactions that are possible, but because of reactions that are barely possible. Too much reactivity and we would spontaneously combust. Too little and we would turn cold and die. Proteins enable these barely possible reactions, allowing us to live on the edges of chemical entropy—skating perilously, but never falling in."

Covid's spike protein doesn't serve any useful function in the body. The sole purpose of the spike is to hook or poke its way inside a cell, where it can hijack the cell's ability to make more of it, lots more of it, to make it "go viral."

Breakthroughs that led to scientists being able to understand the virus's spike protein began in the 1950s. During that decade, researchers first managed to "see" inside the nuclei of cells, and identify the molecules that are the basic building blocks of all life, in the double helix of DNA (an acronym for tongue-twisting deoxyribonucleic acid) and its single-stranded relative in the chemistry of life, RNA (ribonucleic acid).

Once these strands were visualized, it was only a matter of time combined with computer and imaging technology before humans had mapped the linked chain of DNA that is the blueprint of human life, the human genome. Researchers finished the Human Genome Project in April 2003, a landmark in medical history that coincided with the barbarous "shock and awe" beginning of the lie-based, geopolitics-altering Iraq War. Mapping the genome was one of the greatest advances in the history of biology. Its effects on medicine and, really, society are only just beginning to be felt.

Every living thing, including the virus, has a genome. Coiled in each cell, the human genome of DNA, with its precise order of amino acids, is the blueprint for every life.

Straightened out, the human genome would cover two hundred kilometers.

Since the 1950s, researchers made great strides with what came to be known as gene therapy. Besides mapping the human genome, they discovered a way to manipulate it: bacteria living in the geysers of Yellowstone National Park produce an enzyme that they could use to alter genetic material. This breakthrough, known by its acronym CRISPR, dramatically increased the ability of researchers to cut bits of genetic material, essentially molding and shaping genes.

The advent of CRISPR and the new science and practice of gene manipulation have provoked great paranoia in the public and trepidation among scientists themselves. World scientific bodies have tried to maintain order in the new age, forbidding certain types of experiments on human and animal genetics that could alter the forms of life on earth.

Researchers argue that some of these alterations will improve the future. Others—including the vast majority of people who don't work in the field—are suspicious of these claims, to varying degrees. They imagine a dystopia of half-man, half-animal creatures, or the future of the human race altered by generations fed on genetically modified food. Europeans tightly restricted genetically modified organism (GMO) American produce and meat from their markets. Most Americans still consume and feed to their kids cornflakes made with genetically modified corn and burgers made from cows fed with the same.

The Dr. Frankenstein possibilities in genetic engineering haunt the public imagination, but in the labs, where the principle of "experimentation equals progress" prevails, many scientists see endless opportunity. The National Institutes of Health (NIH) has in the past funded so-called gain of function studies, in which researchers manipulate viruses to make them more, not less, communicable and pathogenic, with the aim of beating nature to the dangerous evolutionary moment, and preparing antidotes.

THE MESSENGER

For eons, humanity has been vexed by pathogenic viruses. In the almost 250 years since the advent of the attenuated virus vaccine, there has been a way to fight back. And the platform was always the same.

Until today.

Viruses are as primal as the chemical soup from which life emerged. Covid is in the same classification as two other recently emerged deadly human coronaviruses, MERS and SARS.

All three are believed to have emerged from bats.

In 1961, researchers discovered a substance they called messenger RNA (mRNA). This transient form of RNA carries genetic instructions from the DNA itself to ribosomes (the protein-making factories of the cell). Its simple chemical makeup operates like a code, with instructions to the cell about how to assemble amino acids to make specific proteins. By the 1970s, researchers believed that mRNA might become the platform for a new kind of medicine, delivering genetic instructions synthesized in the lab directly into cells so that the body itself could produce disease-fighting drugs. At the Massachusetts Institute of Technology, a bioengineer named Robert Langer led the first successful effort to encapsulate mRNA strands in lipid nanoparticles, enabling them to enter the body and do their work without being broken down by enzymes. Once inside the body, it was thought, synthetic mRNA could target a multi-tude of illnesses, including cancer.

But what worked in the petri dish wasn't easy to transfer into the human body. In 1990, researchers pulled off the first in vivo test of mRNA in animals (mice). In 2008, a company called Shire Pharmaceuticals began working on mRNA therapies for people with cystic fibrosis.

It wasn't until 2018 that the FDA approved the first lipid nanoparticle carrier for a cancer fighter called siRNA. Unlike mRNA, siRNA "silences" its target—mutated genes.

As Covid emerged in Wuhan, China, in late 2019, micro-biologists and their backers in the pharma industry already understood that humanity was on the cusp of a new kind of medicine. It just needed testing. Investors were already putting it to work on rare diseases and cancers. The attenuated virus vaccine of the English milkmaid and the cowpox worked, but it was analog compared to the digital promise of synthesized atomic biology.

Synthetic mRNA is faster to make, a lot faster: it can be produced in a matter of hours compared to weeks or months fermenting or growing attenuated virus. It is also safer. And, since the synthetic RNA is not a pathogen, large-scale manufac-turing labs don't require the strict and cumbersome advanced biosafety protocols.

Microbiologists knew all of this. A few companies had been making small experimental batches of therapeutic mRNA—a broader class of medicine than vaccines. A few clinical trials were wending their slow way through the experimental "valley of death"—a waiting period required by cautious regulators. None of it was approved. They had been waiting for a "go" signal.

That green light suddenly flashed on January 10, 2020. As an untold number of people in Wuhan staggered into emergency rooms, turning blue, their blood clotting, their organs failing, Chinese scientists posted the genetic sequence of the Covid virus online. Three days later, across the planet, American researchers designed the first mRNA vaccine to counter the new virus.

The earthquake of the pandemic was soon rocking every corner of the planet. A tsunami of money would follow.

CHAPTER 3

The Race

We have been waiting and hoping for the day when the searchlights of science would pick out our invisible enemy and give us the power to stop that enemy from making us ill. And now the scientists have done it, and they have used the virus itself to perform a kind of biological jiu-jitsu, to turn the virus on itself in the form of a vaccine.

—PRIME MINISTER BORIS JOHNSON
announcing UK approval of the first Covid vaccine,
December 2, 2020

Science is the belief in the ignorance of experts.

—RICHARD FEYNMAN

A PEPTO-BISMOL PINK BAG OF WHITE BLOOD CELLS

Seattle, June 4, 2020, 9 a.m.

Missy Peña reclined on a gurney with two giant needles jammed into her inner arms. At thirty-three and in perfect health, she had gotten used to regular blood draws as one of the first forty-five Covid vaccine trial participants in the world. But this draw at the Washington Center for Apheresis Therapy was on a whole other level, with a humming biotech vampire machine attached to her. She tried not to jostle the iPad in her lap, which had *Avatar* cued up. It was her favorite movie, and she never got tired of it; today it was helping her ignore the sound of her blood bubbling out of her body and back in.

The giant needles were connected to clear plastic tubes that were attached to a large plastic box called an apheresis machine. The machine suctioned Peña's blood out of one arm, sifted and captured white blood cells, and then returned the blood back into her other arm. For four hours, Peña lay still as the machine collected her white blood cells.

The vegan illustrator was now also a medical milestone, one of the first humans ever to receive an mRNA vaccine.

Until Covid hit, Peña had little interest in medical news. She sold her fantasy- and gamer-themed artwork at comic book and science fiction conventions around the country. She learned of the Covid vaccine trial by chance via a Twitter notice around March 3, a time when for most Americans the coronavirus was still only faraway news, albeit increasingly alarming. Peña had been more affected than most. She lived in Seattle, where the first US Covid death had been announced. And the conventions where she made her living kept getting canceled. She had just flown back from her last one in Chicago, and was so stressed out about the virus that she had worn a mask on the plane.

She clicked on the link, read the brief notice seeking forty-five participants for an NIH Division of Microbiology and Infectious Diseases "Phase I, Open-Label, Dose-Ranging Study of the Safety and Immunogenicity of 2019-nCoV Vaccine (mRNA-1273) in Healthy Adults." The address for the clinical trials was at a Kaiser Permanente location not far from her home. She decided to apply.

Clinical trials of new vaccines run in three phases. Phase one is primarily concerned with safety, and phase two adds in placebos. These first two phases are conducted on small groups of people. The third phase involves much larger numbers of people, and includes placebo shots as a control. The first phase is theoretically the most dangerous. Animal studies—which precede human trials—can only go so far in predicting how the human body will react. Trial participants must agree to the risks.

Three days after she filled out the form, Peña got a call and an email with the first of dozens of consent forms to read and sign. The consent form informed her that the mRNA-1273 vaccine "has shown promise in animal models, and this is the first trial to examine it in humans." It warned her that the risks included death and unknown long-term effects. Throughout the trial, Peña said, the clinicians never stopped reminding her of the risks, asking if she was sure she wanted to continue.

"I just had to help," Peña said. "Both of my parents and my grandfather were firefighters. I don't come from a science background but my family are about self-sacrifice. And as an artist I feel like I have a very selfish career. I do what I love, and it doesn't feel like work."

On Saint Patrick's Day, Peña received the first shot. The clinical trial had divided participants into groups of fifteen, giving each a different dose. She has never been told her dosage. They sent her home with a thermometer and a soft ruler, for measuring her temperature and any arm swelling. The injection site was moderately sore for three days. Three weeks later, she got her second dose, and that one did cause a night of chills, fatigue, and low fever.

She returned for weekly blood draws, and in May submitted to the leukapheresis (so named because *leuko* means "white," as in leukocytes, or white blood cells), a step further in the trial that not all the participants had agreed to. Peña was allowing researchers to cycle all her blood through a machine for four hours to see how and whether the vaccine had made her body more Covid-proof.

When she glanced away from her iPad, she could see a clear plastic bag attached to the humming machine, slowly filling up with a weird Pepto-Bismol pink liquid. It was gross and fascinating at the same time. These were her white blood cells, separated from her blood by the machine for easier study.

Peña said she was happy to do it, even though the sacrifices continue today. In fall, she found a new job in Barcelona, working for a Spanish gaming company. But she had committed to regular blood draws for fourteen months after the first shot, so she remains in Seattle. She's scheduled to move to Barcelona later. Vials of her blood, and her fully sequenced genome, will remain back at home with American scientists for future study.

When she signed on, Peña knew she was involved in an important public health event. But she didn't know that the vaccine that made her arm sore and gave her a slight fever was destined to be mass-produced and given to millions of Americans—the beginning of the long-awaited "genetic plug and play," as vaccinologist Dr. Paul Offit put it. For the first time outside the lab, medical science was dipping into the primordial soup of life, picking out strands of RNA floating in the salty nano-sea of cell nuclei, and turning the human body into its own drug factory.

THE EDISON OF MEDICINE

Across the continent in Cambridge, Massachusetts, while Peña and forty-four other souls were getting the first shots of the experimental vaccine, a celebrated Massachusetts Institute of Technology chemical engineer was paying keen attention. In his early seventies, Robert Langer was about to be told that the university would not allow him to do any more in-person lectures, due to the incipient danger of the Covid virus. He was healthy, but statistics put him well into the severe Covid danger zone. That was not why he was alert to the doings in Seattle, though.

Langer is a cofounder of the company that made the vaccine injected into Peña's arm. Long before the pandemic, as an obscure young researcher, he had played a role in the research that made the vaccine possible. In the 1970s, he was among a tiny group of chemists trying to coax mRNA into becoming a medical tool. Langer discovered that by encasing mRNA strands in tiny blobs of fat, they could elude enzymes in the body that would otherwise wipe them out before they reached cells. That particular discovery sat on the shelf for decades, because no one could figure out how to trick the body's immune system into not overreacting. Langer couldn't get funding to proceed and he moved on.

Sometimes called the Edison of medicine, Langer has patented or has patents pending on fourteen hundred discoveries, and he's teamed with venture capitalists and pharmaceutical companies to bring those discoveries to patients. He heads the biggest biomedical engineering lab in the world, the Langer Lab at the Massachusetts Institute of Technology's Department of Chemical Engineering. The lab employs one hundred researchers (most university labs employ ten to twenty-five maximum) and rakes in millions annually in grant funding.

Langer's greatest discoveries have to do with noninvasive methods of delivering medication or extracting information from the body. Among his inventions is a wafer that can be implanted in the brain to deliver chemotherapy directly to the site of a tumor, and a potential cure for type 1 diabetes that, like the mRNA invention does but on the cellular level, encases therapeutic but foreign cells in polymer to protect them from the body's immune reaction.

Many more of Langer's discoveries are still in the pipeline. One of the venture capitalists that has backed discoveries from his lab believes that, in sum total, his lab's inventions have the potential to affect nearly 4.7 billion lives.

In 2010, a venture capitalist approached Langer. Other researchers had finally moved the ball on mRNA and found ways to get it into the body. With the financers, Langer founded Moderna (named after modulated RNA itself).

As Langer's own experience with mRNA shows, scientists can wait decades after a promising discovery to the first human test. In pharmaceuticals, long time frames are the norm. Far more discoveries don't even get to the first human trial than become licensed for use.

In the world of medical testing, the Covid vaccine set a land speed record. The Chinese put the new virus genome online on January 10. Three days later—and still twenty-seven days before the WHO declared a national emergency—the NIH and Moderna were running experiments on ways to manipulate the coronavirus's spike protein. By early February—a month before the first known Covid death in the United States—they had designed an mRNA vaccine, and were watching immunized mice develop antibodies against the coronavirus's spike protein.

A month later, Peña and forty-four others were signing up to get their first shots.

The vaccine manufacturer Moderna is a small, sleek, and very well-financed company. When Covid hit, Moderna employed only eight hundred people, including a manufacturing team. In 2019, it had twenty vaccines and treatments in development. It hadn't sold a single one and none were expected to come to market for at least two years. It had never run a phase three clinical trial to determine whether a vaccine is safe and effective for large numbers of humans.

Moderna was formed on a grand possibility: that mRNA was on the cusp of being a tool for myriad therapeutics. The odds were slim, but the potential payoff in both money and life-saving medicine could be staggering. Moderna's CEO, Stéphane Bancel, a former salesman, left a much bigger pharmaceutical firm to join the company in 2011. At the time, Bancel estimated that the mRNA method had a 5 percent chance of success. But if it did succeed, he told his wife at the time, it would change the course of modern medicine. Investors thought so too. The company went public in 2018 with the largest biotech initial public offering in history.

The research that led to the first mRNA vaccine represents the peak of a series of technological and intellectual advances that, one could argue, began in the early eighteenth century, with the Dutch businessman Antonie van Leeuwenhoek. An avid amateur experimenter, he spent his life grinding ever more specialized lenses that eventually allowed human eyes to see microbes for the first time. In the centuries since, technology has enabled human eyes to see ever tinier and tinier creatures until finally peering into the filaments that are the core of all life.

By the time the pandemic hit, researchers not only knew the code for the virus's RNA, they could also synthesize mRNA in laboratories within days. They could even mass-produce it.

The manufacturing process begins with combining chemicals and biological molecules in test tubes to synthesize and then purify the mRNA. Robots are involved: adding, mixing, heating, and filtering reagents. Machines combine the liquid containing the mRNA in a test tube with a cocktail of different lipids, including natural cholesterol, and a chemical called polyethylene glycol, or PEG. Since lipids are insoluble, they aggregate into nanoparticles, encapsulating the strands of RNA—similar to how enteric aspirin or other coated pills assist the delivery of medicines into the body.

HALL OF HEROES

> *Think through and then at the end of it, you have to say,*
> *"What can I do?" Because then you don't waste your life.*
>
> —KATALIN KARIKÓ

Coronaviruses were first observed during the mid-1930s, and first documented in a human suffering from a cold in 1960. In 2002 and again in 2012, zoonotic "spillover" coronaviruses (literally, viruses spilling over in evolutionary terms, from animal to human pathogens) appeared in Asia and the Middle East, under the names SARS (severe acute respiratory syndrome) and then MERS (Middle East respiratory syndrome). These diseases were deadlier than Covid but not nearly as contagious. All of them appear to have originated in bats.

Years before the Covid virus jumped from bat to man and evolved into a brain-corroding, blood-congealing, oxygen-starving human infection, years before Chinese scientists sequenced this new monster's genome, before the death race between states competing for ventilators and the horrific daily death curves, before the billions and the biotech stock windfalls, before the military airlifts and the first fleets of trucks rolled out loaded with ultra-cold packages destined for the first of hundreds of millions of arms, years before all that, there were the researchers, increasing the sum of human knowledge mostly by infinitesimal steps.

A legion of postdocs were living on takeout Starbucks in their white coats, toiling year after year in sterile labs, doing highly specialized work, sharing and studying each other's work, speaking a language unknown to outsiders but understood within their small circle of genetic medicine scientists, writing grant after grant after grant to keep their work going for another year.

One of these worker bees was a Hungarian biochemist named Katalin Karikó. She was born behind the Iron Curtain in 1955 in Hungary, and studied biochemistry in Soviet-era Budapest. In 1985, she fled Eastern Europe with cash stuffed in her daughter's teddy bear, moved to Pennsylvania, and focused on what was then a backwater in genetic medicine. Biochemists thought mRNA could be used to turn human cells into their own drug treatment factories. But it remained just a theory for decades. No one had made it past the first hurdle of tricking the body into accepting the synthetic strands of genetic material. Time and again they tried, and time and again severe immune reactions wiped out lab animals.

The field was such a dead end that the University of Pennsylvania demoted Karikó because she failed to maintain a stream of grant money to fund her work. A downgrade from her tenure track position to researcher was a professional and financial disaster for her. "I was up for promotion, and then they just demoted me and expected that I would walk out the door," she said. Karikó sucked up her pride and took the lower-paying job in order to keep her green card and maintain coverage for her daughter's college tuition as a Penn employee. It was a low point in her life and career, but "I just thought . . . you know, the [lab] bench is here, I just have to do better experiments," she said.

Karikó persevered, and two decades later, she and another Penn researcher, Drew Weissman, discovered a way to trick the body into letting the messenger into its cells. When the mRNA vaccine went into human arms, it was thanks in large part to their research.

While Karikó was working with mRNA in Pennsylvania, just a state away, in Bethesda, Maryland, another researcher toiled in obscurity. Dr. Barney Graham, the deputy director of the Vaccine Research Center and chief of the Viral Pathogenesis Laboratory at the NIH, had devoted much of his career to the study of a childhood respiratory infection, RSV, that annually sends fifty-seven thousand US kids to the hospital and sometimes kills them.

Like the coronavirus, RSV had a protein that stabbed its way into cells. Also like the coronavirus's spike protein, the RSV's protein shape-shifted in the process of infecting cells, making it especially difficult to control. In 2013, Dr. Graham and his team were able to solve the problem, enabled by advances in technology like X-ray crystallography and cryo-electron microscopy that allowed for high, near-atomic resolution (on the order of one billionth of a meter) visualization of protein structures. They understood that viral proteins change shape once they are inside cells, and they devised a molecular stabilization tool to help cells recognize a viral protein before it entered and morphed into a new form.

Altogether, Langer's and other researchers' early work on the lipid encasement of the protein, Karikó and Weissman's mRNA work, and the NIH team's new viral protein-stabilization tool enabled the creation of an entirely new class of vaccine—the one now aimed at controlling the Covid pandemic.

The final element was money.

The biotech bubble was expanding in 2005, when Karikó and Weissman's paper first attracted the attention of entrepreneurs sniffing around for discovery. Besides Langer, and the venture capital founders of Moderna, a German husband-and-wife team of scientists took notice. Ugur Sahin was born in Iskenderun, Turkey, and raised in Cologne, Germany, where his parents worked at a Ford factory. While working on his doctorate, he met Özlem Türeci, also the daughter of Turkish immigrants. The couple were so devoted to cancer research that on the day they were married, Sahin and Türeci returned to the lab.

In 2001, Sahin and Türeci founded Ganymed Pharmaceuticals, developing drugs to treat cancer using monoclonal antibodies. After Karikó and Weissman's paper was published, Sahin and Türeci founded another company, BioNTech, to harness mRNA to treat cancer. Karikó signed on as a senior vice president. BioNTech's mRNA work positioned it as a prime candidate when Pfizer went looking for a Covid mRNA vaccine.

Today the two doctors are billionaires, among Germany's richest people. They sold Ganymed in 2016 for $1.4 billion. They reportedly still ride their bicycles to work from the modest apartment they share with their daughter. They do not own a car.

STAR TREK AND THE LABRADOODLE BREEDER

*If we can develop an atomic bomb in
2.5 years and put a man on the moon in seven years,
we can do this this year, in 2020.*

—HHS SECRETARY ALEX AZAR

The administration was stumbling. Politics was drowning out science, the experts were being sidelined. The virus was burning through New York City. The president was holding ad hoc evening press briefings promoting quack cures and issuing lying bromides about tests and numbers, disputed in real time even as they fell from his lips. To top it off, the *Wall Street Journal* had just revealed something astonishing about a young political protégé in charge of the day-to-day Covid response. Brian Harrison, thirty-seven, had started out as a confidential assistant to Alex Azar and worked his way up to chief of staff. His only prior business experience was operating a dog-breeding company called Dallas Labradoodles.

Yes. A dog breeder was running the nation's early day-to-day Covid response.

Azar is a man who can withstand a great deal of public humiliation—that much was evident in his toadying appearances at the nightly press conferences. He was being crushed between the truth sayers in the science and medical community under his domain and his magical-thinking big boss. And like so many of his colleagues in the Trumpian public health policy pantheon, he was deeply religious, which affected his views on science in very fundamental ways.

On the weekend after the *Wall Street Journal* revealed that his friend the dog breeder was running the pandemic response,

Azar took a long walk around Washington to cool his head. An idea came to him, a bolt from the Guy in the Sky maybe. A big idea. Redemption for him. He called it a "big hairy audacious goal or BHAG" in the MBA-speak Trumpies favored. The administration would uncap a Niagara Falls of federal money, billions and billions, on pharmaceutical companies willing to test and manufacture vaccines simultaneously. If the vaccines didn't work, the companies would still get paid. Money talks, bullshit walks. Now no one could accuse them of not taking the "hoax" seriously enough.

A government bypass was needed. A small group of industry-associated advisers would choose the most promising vaccine and therapeutics research at the companies most able to mass-produce it.

Silo it off from oversight and regulations.

And hit "go."

The president liked the sound of this. He liked it even more when an FDA oncologist and *Star Trek* fan involved in formulating the new effort came up with the name "Operation Warp Speed." That had just the right Hollywood ring. On *Star Trek*, "warp" refers to the highest drive speed on the starship *Enterprise*. When engaged, the ship would blow through millions of light-years by "warping" space-time.

OWS, as it came to be known, would boldly go where no man had gone before, just like Captain Kirk and the starship *Enterprise*.

In June, the new OWS website premiered online, with the promise to "produce and deliver 300 million doses of safe and effective vaccines with the initial doses available by January 2021."

This was indeed the promise of a medical research warp speed at which no man had gone before. And no man would.

Until the pandemic, neither BioNTech nor Moderna had managed to license a single mRNA project. They had neither persuaded regulators to grant human trials, nor convinced them that the challenges the therapies faced were big or urgent enough to warrant expedited study.

Sometimes nature took care of the diseases the projects were designed to combat before vaccines could be tested. Experimental vaccines for SARS, MERS, and Zika didn't get to large clinical trials because those epidemics had died down by the time vaccines were ready for testing.

That sleepy pace changed in a period of weeks. In the first half of April, as funeral homes and morgues were overwhelmed, two dozen bodies a day were being buried on Hart Island in the Bronx, and a city official suggested burying overflow Covid corpses in temporary trenches in New York parks. The NIH drafted and approved a new set of rules by which to rapidly test experimental Covid vaccines. An advisory group drafted a single unified data and safety board for all the trials.

OWS would be a public-private partnership, staffed with pharmaceutical industry insiders and scientists and civil servants from various government agencies including the CDC, HHS, the NIH, BARDA, and the Department of Defense (DoD). The team took up residence on two floors in the Hubert H. Humphrey Building on Independence Avenue in Washington, DC—HHS offices but with a decidedly Pentagon flavor. A preponderance of the government staff showed up in uniforms. The top staff consulted a tome called *Freedom's Forge*, about American military-industrial collaboration during World War II, and scheduled their meetings according to a "battle rhythm" starting at 8 a.m.

Former Big Pharma executive Moncef Slaoui, Euro-soigné,

was tapped to oversee the scientific side—approving funding and coordinating vaccine and therapeutics research. Army general Gustave "Gus" Perna was responsible for security, supply, production, and distribution. Both men would end up having to explain themselves: Slaoui for his Moderna stock share windfalls and for keeping half a million shares of his former employer, Glaxo Smith Kline, even as he oversaw the awarding of $2 billion in taxpayer money to the pharma giant, and Perna for what would prove to be epic failures in supply and distribution once the vaccines were approved.

Before OWS was formed, vaccines had already been injected into thousands of test subjects like Missy Peña. Moderna was well into its phase two trials. Pfizer, partnered with BioNTech, had produced twenty candidate mRNA vaccines by March 11, the day WHO declared Covid a pandemic. During the next month, BioNTech tested its prototype vaccines on mice, rats, and monkeys, and then on its first humans in Germany. It injected its first vaccine into American human arms six weeks after Moderna's first Seattle trial.

OWS ultimately spent $18 billion, mostly on six pharmaceutical companies to develop six different vaccines. The companies were attracted by guaranteed money. Whether or not the vaccines worked, the government would pay for research and simultaneous testing and manufacturing. They also got other assurances, chiefly a blanket release from legal liability if the vaccines hurt anyone.

Throughout spring and summer, hundreds of thousands of people signed up as human guinea pigs for a Covid shot or a placebo. None died or suffered what were considered dangerous side effects. Unique in modern American pharmaceutical history, this was a true warp-speed event. In normal times, some clinical trials can take fifteen years. They constituted a risky, costly challenge that had deterred companies from vaccine research in favor of research that was more lucrative. Only the best funded and most tested medicines made it across the so-called valley of death. Previous mRNA vaccines and many other medical innovations lingered as ghostly residents in that final phase for years before they could apply for a license.

The first decision was which vaccine candidates to back, out of almost fifty possible contenders. Slaoui's team decided to back three types of vaccine platforms. The first was the mRNA platform, in which mRNA containing instructions for how to make the coronavirus's spike protein is packaged into fat droplets for delivery to our cells. The second was the viral vector platform, in which the instructions are encoded in DNA instead of mRNA, and the vehicle for delivery is a non-infectious adenovirus that has been modified to be incapable of replication. The third was a protein-based platform, in which a modified (recombinant) version of the coronavirus's spike protein is synthesized in the lab and delivered directly to the patient.

Each platform was to be pursued by two companies, in case one firm failed. Federal officials referred to the finalists as "horses," a nod to the race between them. The six companies were Moderna and Pfizer/BioNTech (both mRNA), AstraZeneca and Johnson & Johnson (both viral vector), and Novavax and Sanofi/GSK (recombinant). (Pfizer declined the federal OWS money but signed a $2 billion contract to sell vaccines to the US government later in summer 2020.)

Critics complained that the decision making behind the selection process was opaque and the announcement came without explanation. "It's been so chaotic, and it's not even transparent to those of us who are trying to help out," a Warp Speed source who asked not to be named told *Science* magazine at the time.

The new platform is a medical milestone. It will probably bring new tools to fight other emergent diseases, as well as cancer. It is doubtful this would have happened without the mother's milk of the American health care system.

Money.

OF MICE AND MEN AND MONEY

I have never been about the money, ever.

—MONCEF SLAOUI, head of Operation Warp Speed

Big Pharma had been easing out of the vaccine business for decades. By 2019, the major vaccine makers supplying America had dwindled to a handful of large companies—Merck, Sanofi, Pfizer, and Johnson & Johnson. Because vaccines are only used once or twice—as opposed to medicines that people take daily—they are not profitable. The scale of vaccination programs also invites class action litigation if something goes awry.

The White House needed a whopping amount of money to coax companies to research and test and then produce hundreds of millions of doses. They initially asked for and Congress rapidly appropriated $10 billion. Ultimately OWS would dole out $22 billion to Big Pharma.

The amounts of money were the kinds of sums normally seen in the smaller defense budget line items, but were massive for a public health project—$2.5 billion to Moderna, $1.2 billion to AstraZeneca, half a billion dollars to Johnson & Johnson, and $1.6 billion to a small company called Novavax. Only Pfizer opted out of ponying up to the trough at first—it didn't want to devote resources to coordinating with the US government on its work. In July, Pfizer signed a $1.95 billion deal to sell one hundred million doses of its two-shot vaccine to the United States, enough for fifty million people. It would be the first to reach American arms. The price per double shot—about forty dollars—is comparable to the price per shot of the flu vaccine. By February, the government had ordered three hundred million doses from Moderna, with its first shipment of one hundred million priced at thirty dollars per double-shot dose—cheaper than Pfizer partly because the United States had forked over nearly a billion dollars to Moderna research. Moderna's CEO has said the price per dose will be higher for retail once the government contracts phase out.

Because the project worked, it may well elude financial investigation.

OWS was staffed at every level by pharmaceutical industry executives and their revolving door of allies in the government. They could, if they wished, keep their investments thanks to a special exemption. Brought on as "contractors," they were not subject to federal conflict-of-interest regulations in place for employees. OWS advisers with connections and investments had to agree to assign some of their Covid vaccine earnings to the NIH—but they could wait to do so until after their deaths.

Slaoui sat on the board of Moderna. Thirteen days after the first massive infusion of taxpayer money into its coffers—which triggered a jump in the company's stock price—Slaoui was awarded options to buy 18,270 shares in the company, according to Securities and Exchange Commission filings first reviewed by Kaiser Health News. Those shares were added to 137,168 options he'd accumulated since 2018. He reaped an estimated $8 million when he resigned from the Moderna board.

Among the other known connections between OWS and Big Pharma cash: OWS advisers and Pfizer employees William Erhardt and Rachel Harrigan maintained financial stakes of unknown value in Pfizer, the recipient of a nearly $2 billion HHS contract for one hundred million doses of its vaccine. Richard Whitley, an adviser on the vaccine safety panel, is associated with Gilead, maker of the Covid antiviral agent remdesivir. Adviser Carlo de Notaristefani is connected to Teva, maker of the Trump-approved hydroxychloroquine. Former FDA commissioners Dr. Scott Gottlieb and Dr. Mark McClellan, informally advising the federal response, both have seats on the boards of Covid vaccine developers.

Slaoui eventually issued a vague threat about criticism of the insiders' big gains. The media focus on his and other OWS advisers' profits might delay the vaccine, he suggested in a podcast "interview" with HHS communications director Michael Caputo. (Caputo, we recall, would tell Facebook followers that the medical deep state was going to prevent a timely vaccine and to arm up before the election, then resign after blaming his bizarre social media rants on mental issues.)

"I'm amazed that I'm being attacked on a personal basis in a way that frankly distracts my energy and the energy of all the teams we're working together with to deliver, and therefore decreases our chances or the speed with which we try to help humanity and the country resolve and address this issue," Slaoui said.

Unlike Caputo and Azar at HHS, Slaoui was no political hack. He never toadied to Trump and did not accelerate or pressure vaccine makers to meet Trump's blatantly political goal of a vaccine before the November election. He also vowed to donate any money he earned on his company stocks while in his post to research.

Even more money was raining down on company insiders trading on good-news releases. Executives at Moderna and Pfizer cashed in on the vaccine, selling shares timed precisely to clinical trial press releases.

Timing stock sales like that is neither unusual nor illegal. Columbia Law School economist Joshua Mitts has found that execs in many sectors are up to three times more likely to sell off their company stock on days when their companies announce positive news than on days when negative, neutral, or no news is released.

On November 9, the day Pfizer announced its more than 90 percent vaccine efficacy, Pfizer CEO Albert Bourla sold more than half of his holdings—62 percent. It was a good day to sell—the positive news jacked stock prices 15 percent. Bourla was among seven Pfizer executives who collectively earned $14 million from stock sales in 2020, according to data provided to the *Los Angeles Times* by Equilar, an executive compensation and corporate governance data firm.

Not to be outdone, Moderna executives made $287 million from timed stock sales in 2020—and kept going. In just a few days in late January and February 2021, Moderna CEO Stéphane Bancel sold millions of dollars' worth of his stock.

The Trump administration's best and brightest Covid solution—throw public money at private industry with almost no oversight of the contracting procedure—will stand as one of the most audacious efforts in the administration's free market ideological playbook. The full roster of this pharmaceutical windfall club will probably never be revealed. The Pandemic Response Accountability Committee, established through the first Covid relief bill (the CARES Act), is an independent body assigned to track the $2.6 trillion appropriated in government funds to deal with the crisis, but it has its mandate focused on the funds spent on the recovery, not the vaccine.

As public policy, OWS paid off in one big way: three unexpectedly effective vaccines went from concept to human arms in less than a year.

In other ways, OWS did not deliver. A warp-speed project on therapeutics might have prevented some of the more than half a million American deaths.

The pandemic crisis offered a challenge that government might have used to restructure the shareholder model of for-profit medicine, a model that dates to the 1980s and corporate America's turn toward putting shareholders above the public good. Instead, taxpayer money flowed to a small group of capitalists with almost no strings attached and little transparency. The contracts are redacted, although Freedom of Information Act (FOIA) requests are pending.

As cities across the nation started vaccinating at the end of 2020, the media sought out and hailed some of the researchers as heroes. And they are heroes. But most researchers would not cash in. The NIH's Barney Graham, whose work on molecular protein manipulation is key to the Moderna vaccine, gets paid a government salary. Moderna execs, besides pocketing nearly a billion dollars, will still charge Americans for its vaccine. Katalin Karikó is on the board at BioNTech, but—as per common practice in the world of medical research—she doesn't hold the patent for her discovery; the University of Pennsylvania does.

MEDICAL MILESTONE

Two days after Trump officially lost the presidential election to Joe Biden on November 7, Pfizer announced that its phase three clinical trials were complete and its vaccine was more than 90 percent effective. Six days later, Moderna announced its trials were concluded. Shortly after that, the FDA—the same FDA that had refused to allow the foreign WHO tests in the United States, and then refused to allow non-CDC tests to supplement the CDC's flawed test at the beginning of the pandemic—gave Pfizer and Moderna "emergency use" approval.

This good news came just weeks too late for Trump to take credit.

Trump "fumed," "raged," and "lashed out" when Pfizer announced the stunning vaccine efficacy two days after Joe Biden "stole" the election from him. The timing confirmed his and his political health agency appointees' paranoid suspicion that even Big Pharma—the very companies they had lavished with no-bid contracts—was conspiring against his reelection.

Trump might have gone truly mad had he been informed of the actual reason for the delay: Moderna, first out of the gate with its clinical tests in March, should have reached the finish line a bit earlier. But it hit a roadblock that Pfizer—which had declined OWS funding to avoid government involvement in its work—did not have to reckon with. In August, OWS's Slaoui informed Moderna that it had not recruited enough minority candidates into its vaccine trials to meet government require-ments. If it could not prove its vaccine worked as well for Black and Hispanic Americans, groups disproportionately affected by the pandemic in the United States, Moderna's trial would not make it over the finish line.

To comply with the diversity requirement, the company

revised its plan, recruited more people to its trials, and set its timeline back weeks. (Pfizer ended up having the same percentage of Black participants as Moderna, without US government involvement.)

The Pfizer and Moderna results exceeded all expectations. Most vaccines have an average success rate of in the 70s or 80s. The Moderna and Pfizer trials yielded results of more than 90 percent efficacy. "I describe myself as a realist, but I'm fundamentally a cautious optimist," Dr. Fauci told the *Washington Post* after the announcement. "I felt we'd likely get something less than this. . . . I said certainly a 90-plus-percent effective vaccine is possible, but I wasn't counting on it."

Missy Peña's four hours on the gurney hooked up to the apheresis machine in Seattle proved to be an important part of the landmark study. The Pepto-Bismol pink liquid she watched fill the bag confirmed that the mRNA vaccine works in not just one but two ways. Animal studies had shown that the spike protein messenger RNA prompted cells to make antibodies against the spike protein that appeared to neutralize the virus. But the trials showed that the vaccine did something else too: it induced a secondary and deeper immune response, producing T cells that recognize infected cells, and destroy them.

"We've entered a new era, which is this really genetic plug-and-play vaccine era," author and immunization expert Dr. Paul Offit said in an interview, "where you don't inoculate the person with the virus, you inoculate them with a gene that codes for that protein. So you make the protein, your body makes the viral proteins, and your body makes an antibody response to that protein. This is the genetic era. And we'll see to what extent it applies to a variety of other pathogens."

The great irony of this success story is that the project kicked off at the precise point in American history when a clamorous, politically active segment of the American public was most scornful and suspicious of scientists, and our president and his regime were three years into severing the United States from a fact-based, science-run world.

AND THEN THERE WERE DOZENS

In 2020, the US government spent $18 billion on vaccine research, manufacturing, and logistics and approved two for use at the end of the year: the mRNA-platformed Pfizer and Moderna vaccines. The eleven-month concept-to-emergency-approval process set a record in American vaccine history. Nothing else even came close.

Besides the mRNA vaccines, US taxpayers had bet billions on Johnson & Johnson, Novavax, and AstraZeneca, the British company. Johnson & Johnson and AstraZeneca, like the Chinese and Russian vaccine efforts, were making vector vaccines—a newer vaccine model than the attenuated virus model in vogue since the days of the cowpox—using virus modified so that it can enter cells, but cannot replicate itself. The vector vaccines use viruses that the body is familiar with—usually an adenovirus that causes the common cold—to deliver genetic information about specific disease into cells.

In February 2021, Johnson & Johnson reported that its single-shot vaccine, made from an adenovirus carrying Covid spike protein DNA, had a 72 percent efficacy rate. AstraZeneca produced a vaccine also based on a manipulated adenovirus that was already in use in the United Kingdom by February, despite a series of clinical trial mishaps. Novavax, the small Maryland-based company that took $1.6 billion from the US government to produce a protein-based vaccine using material from the soap bark tree as an adjuvant, was bringing up the rear, but promised to have one hundred million doses available in the United States by summer.

By late 2020, a year after Covid showed up in Wuhan, two hundred vaccines were in trials or already in use, according to the WHO—another world record in vaccine history. China's Sinovac was first out of the gate with its inactivated Covid vaccine in June 2020. Another Chinese company, Sinopharm, started tests in the United Arab Emirates, Morocco, and Brazil during summer and made its first sale to the UAE, which began manufacturing it. By early 2021, the UAE was second in the world (behind Israel) in the percentage of its population that had received a vaccination.

The Chinese vaccine dominated the global market, stepping into a soft power vacuum left by US isolationism and pandemic mishaps. By early 2021, three Chinese vaccines were approved and in use, manufactured by Sinovac, Sinopharm, and CanSino—all either based on the adenovirus model or the attenuated Covid virus. In August, Sinovac announced an agreement to sell forty million doses to Indonesia. In February, Hungary became the first European Union country to approve the Sinopharm vaccine for use—after the European Union faced shortages due to the European Commission's inability to cut a deal quickly with vaccine makers in 2020.

In February 2021, the Russian Ministry of Health reported that a vaccine called Sputnik V, based on the vector platform, had a 91.6 percent efficacy rate. Mexico immediately authorized it for use. Canada, Turkey, and South Korea were all testing their own vaccines, and even Cuba had produced a viable vaccine and was reportedly offering it to tourists. Bharat Biotech's inactivated virus vaccine was approved for emergency use in

India. Meanwhile, the Serum Institute of India—the world's largest vaccine-producing factory—was scheduled to manufacture one billion doses of vaccine, mostly for poorer nations.

To be sure, these endeavors did not all meet the standards that Moderna and Pfizer had set. Few in the Western world fully trust official Russian and Chinese numbers about anything. In January 2021, Brazil announced Sinovac's efficacy at 78 percent. A week later, the country revised that to "above 50 percent"—still high enough to meet WHO goals, but the swing from high to merely adequate efficacy nonetheless gives us pause.

Inevitably, the race to the vaccine took on a nationalistic flavor. In August, Russian president Vladimir Putin announced on national state television that Russia's Sputnik V vaccine (named after the USSR's landmark launching of the world's first artificial satellite—plus a "V" for vaccine) was "quite effective," even though it hadn't made it to a phase three trial. The Brits took to calling the Oxford-developed AstraZeneca shot "the English one," and in Germany, Pfizer—which received early German funding—was called "the German one" with pride.

But the challenge also spawned some intriguing collaborations, suggesting that the virus could inspire the notion of a brotherhood of nations and corporations on the fractious planet. Russia and the United Kingdom, for example, announced they were going to pool their adenovirus vaccines into a single vaccine, to see if the combination amplified efficacy. GSK, based in Britain, and the French company Sanofi, usually competitors, joined forces, putting their combined Big Pharma financial and manufacturing capacity behind a vaccine. And, in March 2021, the White House brokered a collaboration to manufacture vaccines between Merck and Johnson & Johnson.

The flurry of research and collaboration has even led to scientists not just talking about but being on the verge of testing a pan-coronavirus vaccine made of nanoparticles studded with corona proteins, which would be effective against all coronaviruses—even the one that causes the common cold.

Imagine a world without the common cold. Can vanquishing death and taxes be far behind?

COCKTAIL HOUR

A number of photographs from the Trump era could become iconic representations of the era. I tend to favor the one with the Easter Bunny, the fake supermodel, and the wannabe Mussolini all together on the White House balcony one spring morning in 2017. Others prefer the president grinning beside elegant candelabra and piles of hundreds of boxes of McDonald's food in the White House State Dining Room, plastic packets of chicken-nugget dipping sauce in silver bowls that Jackie Kennedy might have used.

The image most likely to memorialize the Trump administration's deadly, cavalier attitude toward the pandemic was snapped on October 5, 2020. On that day, the president left Walter Reed hospital after three days of treatment for Covid, walked unaided into the White House, climbed the steps of the South Portico, and removed his black face mask. Chin jutted Il Duce–style, he stood without speaking, his chest heaving as he struggled to breathe and project strength at the same time.

A few hours earlier, he had tweeted from the Walter Reed Medical Center: "Feeling really good! Don't be afraid of Covid. Don't let it dominate your life. We have developed, under the Trump Administration, some really great drugs & knowledge. I feel better than I did 20 years ago!"

By that day, 209,881 Americans had died of Covid. They had been *dominated*. Within three months, the number of American dead would double. Later, it was revealed that Trump was much sicker than his aides and doctors and he had admitted, and that his staff had leaned on the FDA to get him unapproved drugs pronto. The *New York Times* reported that first son-in-law Kushner later told other people testing positive in Trumpland that he could arrange for the same treatment for them.

In any case, it was going to be a special cocktail hour for a special club.

Shortly after Trump stripped his mask for the cameras, New Jersey Republican Chris Christie, who tested positive for Covid on October 3—hardly surprising given his proximity to Trump at a mask-free debate prep session—was hospitalized. Christie, then fifty-eight, was younger than Trump by two decades but even more obese, and asthmatic. Seven days in the ICU later, the former governor was alive and discharged.

Christie and Trump were not the only Covid miracles. In November, Housing and Urban Development secretary Ben Carson, sixty-nine, announced that he had been "desperately ill" with Covid before Trump "cleared me" to get the special cocktail. In December, former New York mayor and Trump election conspiracist Rudy Giuliani—seventy-six, a heavy drinker and smoker of cigars—reported that he had Covid. From his hospital bed a few days later, he crowed that he was getting the same really great drugs the president had gotten, and that he was feeling better than ever. He said that he was receiving "exactly the same" treatment, and that Trump's "doctor sent me here; he talked me into it. The minute I took the cocktail yesterday, I felt 100 percent better. It works very quickly, wow."

"America's Mayor" wasn't embarrassed about his means of access either. "If it wasn't me, I wouldn't have been put in a hospital frankly," Giuliani told WABC radio in New York. "Sometimes when you're a celebrity, they're worried if something happens to you they're going to examine it more carefully, and do everything right."

He cited his recovery as evidence that businesses should fling open their doors because Covid "is a treatable disease."

For those of us watching at home, it was hard to understand how all this was true, as average Americans were dying like flies. What "really great drugs" had raised these four obese and/or geriatric males—with three if not four Covid comorbidities between them—Lazarus-like out of their hospital beds?

When Covid started killing people in China, doctors were terrified. They had battled coronavirus-caused upper-respiratory killers SARS and MERS a decade earlier. No drugs yet existed to cure those diseases, and it soon was clear the same was true of Covid. Available antiviral drugs could sometimes mitigate the symptoms, but only if administered early. Even then, they did not always save lives.

The search for therapeutics was challenging because Covid's assault on the body is mysteriously multifaceted. It took a while for medics to understand that Covid isn't just a respiratory disease. The virus does enter the body via the airways and causes pneumonia. But it also ravages other organs: heart, kidney, liver—it even invades the lining of the brain, causing brain damage or mental illness. Covid gets into the veins and coagulates the blood, rendering it the consistency of Jell-O. It causes heart and circulatory system damage normally associated with strokes and neuroinflammatory diseases.

Operation Warp Speed wasn't just throwing billions of dollars at the vaccine. Its other, less publicized mission was to support research into therapeutics. Could modern medicine come up with an infusion, a pill, a tonic—anything, even NyQuil or Theraflu—to prevent symptoms and death?

In the summer, HHS announced it was giving New York–based Regeneron Pharmaceuticals $450 million to support the large-scale manufacturing of an investigational antiviral antibody treatment it called REGN-COV2. "This agreement is the first of a number of OWS awards to support potential therapeutics all the way through to manufacturing," the HHS press release read. "As part of the manufacturing demonstration project, doses of the medicine will be packaged and ready to ship immediately if clinical trials are successful and FDA grants [emergency use authorization] or licensure."

By the end of the year, a small number of doses had been distributed, but the drug was not in wide use in hospitals. The treatment, which often included a commonly used strong steroid called dexamethasone, had to be administered intravenously, by infusion over four hours. Overwhelmed hospitals with bodies on gurneys in the hallway didn't have time for this. And it appeared to work best on people who tested positive but weren't yet too sick. Without constant testing, most people didn't know they had the virus until they were too far gone for the drugs to reverse their disease.

In the mask-free world around Trump, the president and his friends were tested constantly. The old men were rapidly hooked up to IV infusions of a "cocktail" of rare monoclonal antibodies developed by Eli Lilly and of two monoclonal antibodies developed by Regeneron. The FDA had approved the treatment under emergency use in November for outpatients with "mild to moderate" disease at high risk for progressing to severe disease or for being hospitalized.

Other than those drugs, the best Americans could hope for was that they didn't get sick enough to be hooked up to the cure of last resort—the dreaded ventilator.

For the record, only Christie emerged from his long cocktail hour in the ICU a reformed man. Not wearing masks, he announced, was "a mistake." And then there's Herman Cain, who didn't emerge at all.

AMERICA FIRST

This is the people's vaccine. Federal scientists helped invent it and taxpayers are funding its development. . . . It should belong to humanity.

—PETER MAYBARDUK, director of Public Citizen's Global Access to Medicines Program

American money and many years of American science launched this medical milestone, the synthetic messenger RNA in a vaccine. In terms of vaccines, we have finally left the eighteenth century. America did that. But America did not actually "win" the race to a Covid vaccine. In fact, its "America First" vaccine effort only highlighted the fact that the United States is no longer a nation to which the world looks for leadership.

The Chinese were. The Chinese claimed to have vaccinated hundreds of millions of people before a single shot ever went into an American arm. With nearly 1.5 billion people and teeming cities across a vast land mass, they started vaccinating without waiting for the usual clinical trial period, and got their outbreak under control within months. Their vaccine was on the global market by summer. The Global South was buying it and producing it in its own factories by fall 2020.

A pandemic, by definition, is a planetary event. It was possible to plausibly deny this for only a few weeks after news out of Wuhan in the last days of 2019.

Trump tried mightily to ignore it. For most of the month of January, he suggested it was a hoax and Fox News amplified that word night after night. At the end of January, he said it was "pretty much under control." On March 10, one day before the WHO declared Covid a pandemic, he stated, "It's really working out."

When the US government finally conceded that the world— and us with it—was indeed headed into a pandemic, and the White House declared a national emergency on March 13, the virus was thick in New York City. Unchecked Covid transmission in the dense metropolis was about to produce the first deadly surge of terminally sick people into hospitals, overwhelming medics, and leading to the spectacle of city parks turned into shallow graves.

The administration and its denizens on Fox took great pride in calling the disease "the China virus" while the White House retreated further into isolationism. On April 14, Trump held a press conference, announcing that he was putting the WHO under investigation for helping China cover up the nature of the virus and the extent of its spread until it was too late. "The world depends on the WHO to work with countries to ensure that accurate information about international health threats is shared in a timely manner, and if it's not, to independently tell the world the truth about what is happening," he said. "The WHO failed in this basic duty and must be held accountable. It's time after all of these decades."

The WHO had stumbled, especially on the efficacy of mask wearing. But so had the CDC. The WHO had offered a Covid test to the world in January, a month when Trump was still claiming the virus was a hoax. The Trump administration had declined.

The pandemic wouldn't pull America back on the global team. The nation was retreating from the world effort, going it alone. Riding off into the sunset, Marlboro Man–style.

"Operation Warp Speed has been very active in paying billions of taxpayer money for procurement contracts and thus hoarding access to the very limited supply of vaccines that the whole world needs, but very inactive in making sure that the vaccines on which it puts its hands actually find their way into the arms of the American people," economist William Lazonick wrote in a long article about the self-defeating xenophobia at the heart of this strategy.

Science, like the pandemic, is global. It is a pan-human endeavor, shared across borders. Even during the Cold War, scientists from the United States and the USSR collaborated or communicated on nonmilitary experiments and advances. Patented technology in capitalist countries doesn't belong to the entire planet, but often the knowledge base that enables inventions is universal.

The futility of trying to isolate one of the most scientifically advanced nations in the world from the rest of the planet was obvious. So was the malice behind it. The national government of the richest nation on earth reacted to the pandemic like Lionel Barrymore's angry banker in Frank Capra's *It's a Wonderful Life*, miserable with his miserly hoard.

America's failure to cooperate with the WHO played out on many levels—at the most basic, in terms of research. In 2020, not surprisingly, a blizzard of articles about Covid overwhelmed peer-reviewed journals. *New England Journal of Medicine* editor Edward Campion was receiving forty Covid-related papers a day, and turning them over to virologists with instructions to review them within twenty-four hours. So-called preprints—not peer reviewed—also were published online.

At least two hundred thousand Covid-related papers were published by the end of 2020. Many were mere opinion papers, lacking original data. Scientists followed the money and the attention, rushing to comment without original data, misleading other scientists and the media. It was possible, through most of 2020, to google whether hydroxychloroquine was good as a treatment for Covid and have a 50 percent chance of getting a yes or a no.

One global institution was immune to this infodemic of unfiltered opinion masquerading as science. According to a study of nearly forty thousand policy documents drafted between January and May 2020, the WHO was the organization most resistant to subpar papers.

"A lot of the way that the science is getting into policy documents at the national level is indirect, so it's basically the World Health Organization, say, will write something, drawing out all this latest science, and then other governments will cite this WHO policy document as opposed to citing the science directly," economist Benjamin Jones, who directed the study, writes. "We see that the places like the WHO, which of course has been pilloried by some political actors in this pandemic, clearly play a very central role. They really are the center of that whole network drawing science into policy."

While the United States looked away from this network and inward, other nations stepped into the void. Collaborations started. Purchasing pools formed. As vaccine studies and plans for distribution were underway, the United States spurned the vaccine collaboration COVAX, a global initiative co-led by Gavi, the Global Vaccine Alliance, the WHO, and the Coalition for Epidemic Preparedness Innovations (CEPI). COVAX aims to distribute two billion vaccine doses to ninety-two low- and middle-income countries at no more than $3 a dose. Johnson & Johnson is working with COVAX, with its one-shot vaccine being distributed by UNICEF.

The essence of the COVAX endeavor, which involved at least 172 nations and eighteen vaccine efforts, was "pooled procurement." Coming together as one amplified the buying power of individual nations and made research and vaccines more affordable. Pooled procurement, to free market ideologues, strips the seller of his or her right to charge what the market will bear. Antagonism to the concept of pooled procurement informed the Trump decision not to make the federal government the sole purchaser of desperately needed equipment, but to force states to compete in the Covid death race.

"Price is always a component" in the Hobbesian Utopia of vulture capital, as Trump sneered at panicked governors in the spring of 2020. "Stronger Together" was never going to be a slogan in MAGA Washington.

As one of his first acts as president, in late January 2021, Biden rejoined the WHO and put the United States into the COVAX partnership. But the damage had already been done.

"I believe that President Trump's decision to cut funding to WHO in the middle of a global pandemic was so egregious that it constituted a crime against humanity," wrote Richard Horton, editor of the British medical journal *Lancet*. "WHO exists to protect the health and wellbeing of the world's peoples. A crime against humanity is a knowing and inhumane attack against a people. By attacking and weakening WHO while the agency was doing all it could to protect individuals in some of the most vulnerable countries in the world, President Trump has, in my view, met the criteria for an act of violence the international community calls a crime against humanity."

TIBERIUS

The researchers, the clinical trial guinea pigs, and the pharmaceutical execs all did their jobs.

Science delivered.

Now the burden of obtaining and distributing three hundred million vaccines fell to the uniformed half of the Operation Warp Speed team. The guys with the stripes and medals on their shoulders.

All summer, the military branch of OWS had done what it could, providing security and greasing the transport of critical machines. When a piece of Moderna factory equipment made in Michigan was delayed en route to Massachusetts because of Covid interstate trucking restrictions, the DoD stepped in. When another piece of critical gear got lost on a train, the OWS logistics team saved the day, grabbing it off the train and putting it on a plane.

But the men from the Pentagon who move aircraft carriers and battalions of war-fighters and matériel from American shores to deserts and jungles overseas proved not up to the task of herding the cats of the broken American health care system. The original idea, as usual in the digital age, was to throw algorithms at the problem and let AI sort it out. IT experts at HHS and the DoD collaborated on a vast data-crunching system. According to the DoD, the program was "a cutting-edge data platform to collect, correlate and visualize data across the entire operation. It is loaded with data from various sources—U.S.

Census, Department of Health and Human Services, State Health Offices and the CDC."

They named it "Tiberius"—not after the first-century Roman emperor known for his martial capabilities, but as a continuation of the *Star Trek* theme: Tiberius was Captain Kirk's middle name.

General Perna announced the program would be "tracking and tracing every dose" because Tiberius would link databases from shipping companies and the government. The first vaccine-loaded trucks emerged from the factory bays on a gray morning in December, with TV cameras recording them, on their way to save lives. It made for stirring television, and it was hard not to get choked up as the first nurse in New York, Sarah Lindsay, held out her arm for the vaccine.

But from there, the snafus started piling up. It was always going to be a problem to deliver vaccines from the freezer farm in Kalamazoo, Michigan, and the distribution center in Pleasant Prairie, Wisconsin, across the country at the ultra-cold temperature required to maintain the stability of the vaccines.

But even with specially designed packages that monitored the temperatures from factory to clinic, the Tiberius databases couldn't reach into the variegated private and public health nooks and crannies of all fifty states.

Meanwhile, the CDC had stepped in with a hierarchy of vaccine-worthy arms, starting with the feeblest in the nursing homes and the frontline medics. Within weeks it was clear that OWS's distribution system wasn't going to meet demand. Like the rest of the chaotic federal approach, delivery would have to be tossed to the states and territories and, from there, to localities.

Things turned *Mad Max*–like practically overnight. If you were connected, you could get it. If not, you were SOL.

At some highly regarded hospitals, from Stanford in California to Columbia in New York, word went out that der-matologists and surgeons and other well-paid staff far from the front lines were getting their first shot, while younger residents who waded into the viral loads and did most of the intubating were at the back of the line.

Most maddening of all, perhaps: mask-less superspreaders in the White House were vaccinated before anyone else.

Almost immediately, the big flaw was obvious. Money and American science had produced a cure for the pandemic. But distrust in government and an atomized polity, engineered and encouraged by the minions creating the Trump regime's Hobbesian Utopia, meant almost nobody could get it.

No one had figured out how to keep track of who got the vaccine. No one had any idea how to make sure people came back for the second shot.

The chaos meant that by the end of 2020, instead of twenty million vaccinated Americans, there were just two million. As the second surge made itself known, and hospitals reached capacity again and dying people spent Christmas and New Year's 2021 on gurneys in hospital hallways again, staffed by nurses and doctors working twelve-hour shifts, seven days a week again, the scientists' triumph didn't mean anything if the logistics team couldn't get it delivered.

The first thing Biden's people did once in the White House was drop the *Star Trek* references. Then they released a two-hundred-page Covid plan, so data-heavy that even experts who had to plow through it were nearly blinded. The message was clear: people who care about facts and listen to science were back in charge in the White House.

CHAPTER 4

Stranger Things
The Mainstreaming of Conspiracy Theory

I think the lay public is fully, fully unprepared
for understanding this.

—KATHERINE O'BRIEN, director of the WHO's
Immunization, Vaccines, and Biologicals program

It's a hoax. There's no pandemic. As
Trump said, how many millions die of flu? If he's
sick, then they planted it when they tested him. It's what
they did to me when I went to hospital for my heart
beating too fast. Two weeks later I got a cold. It's
political. I don't trust the US government at
all. Who are they to mandate personal
safety? I listen to Trump.

—SEAN PATTERSON, Missouri truck driver, October 2020

To date, the origins of SARS-CoV-2 remain
in doubt, and its behavior enigmatic: It has been
reported that "the virus acts like no microbe
humanity has ever seen."

—KARL SIROTKIN and DAN SIROTKIN in a
BioEssays peer-reviewed paper

THE GRAND UNIFYING THEORY

I first encountered the grand unifying theory of the pandemic around a fire pit in a lovely garden on a lush June night in the Midwest. A retired government scientist, a friend of a friend, was holding court on the virus. His former job and his PhD gave him some credibility on the subject, and so we listened.

Covid, he believed, was not what we thought it was. He himself eschewed the mask. The virus wasn't exactly a hoax; it was real. It was just that it was inevitable, and we were powerless against it. And dark human forces were behind it.

Humanity, he pointed out, at its apogee in terms of knowledge and technology, had exhausted the planet's biological limit. Climate change, environmental degradation, the mass extinctions—they all pointed to a bad end.

There was nowhere to hide. No place to go but down.

Covid would kill a lot of us, he predicted.

Even with a vaccine?

He was silent for a bit. The firelight licked the darkness. The stars winked in the black firmament above; lightning bugs flickered in the woods. Our mask-less storyteller had our attention. He knew of what he spoke. Then he started dropping names.

Big names.

Bill Gates. Hillary Clinton. Elon Musk. George Soros. Trump too, sure. All in on it.

Wait, what? Drowsy eyebrows raised in unison. In on *what*?

Well, they all knew something that scientists like him understood pretty well, he said. In order for humanity to survive as a species, the human population would have to decrease by about 80 percent. We needed to get back down to a sustainable number of human beings or the earth was going to fry and turn into Venus. And—well—you must know the elites have a plan.

Elon Musk, Bill Gates, Hillary Clinton, George Soros, European billionaires, Davos people—yeah, maybe even Donald Trump—they had all come to an agreement about what needed to be done.

He wasn't sure about the details of the strategy. Could have been just releasing the virus would be enough. Or maybe it would have something to do with the vaccines that Bill Gates would soon propagate around the world to fight it. *Supposedly fight it.* Maybe all of that, *plus* 5G tracking. Maybe China's ruling party was in on it. Whatever it was, the elites would be among the 20 percent who keep the human species alive on a happier, healthier, human-cleansed planet earth. The rest of us, well. Carpe diem. Enjoy the June night and the firelight.

In the next few weeks, as I traveled around the Midwest, I heard some version of that theory from an astounding number of people. The heartland had been visited by an epidemic of disinformation. There were slight variations: The virus was a hoax and a political weapon to destroy the economy. Hospitals were being paid to inflate Covid death numbers. Any vaccine would contain tracking microchips. 5G had created the virus. The virus was a bioweapon. The coming vaccine was a bioweapon too. Masks made people sick.

You could, if you wanted, mix and match any of these theories, and still find someone who believed in the combination.

The Covid conspiracy infodemic, first, speaks to the enduring lure of superstition in our secular time. Just as science's leaps seemed to herald the twilight of religion and superstition, the human tendency toward conspiracy theory to make sense of the randomness of existence had only increased. The pandemic revealed that the urge toward magical thinking is a vestigial instinct, as powerful as it was in epidemics of yore, from the plague of Athens in antiquity, to the Black Death in the Middle Ages, to the bubonic plague in London in 1666.

In those blind days, before our microbial awareness, there were always comets in the sky, or mad blind soothsayers in the street, who, in retrospect, everyone said had presaged the disaster. In the millennia before the microscope, epidemics were believed to be the work of the gods or sorcerers who visited disease upon the guilty, taking down innocent as collateral damage. Cranks and quacks and conspiracy theorists hung out shingles and took money to advise Londoners in Daniel Defoe's *A Journal of the Plague Year*. People were told to pin dead toads to their collars and pay heed to the predictions of astrologers before stepping outside.

Beliefs about disease are always in the end intensely personal. In the nineteenth century, medical science hadn't come up with the germ theory yet. There was intense controversy around what caused cholera, one of the signature infectious diseases in Western Europe at the time. "Scientists debated about whether cholera was caused by bad air, so essentially the poisonous exhalations of the earth or by a contagious particle which had not been totally defined," medical anthropologist Martha Louise Lincoln said. "But everybody, all the social classes, everybody in their own sort of social niche had a sense of a folk explanation for what caused that disease and what it meant."

Modern medical knowledge never eradicated the folk tradition. And global communications amplified it. The internet era and its algorithms favor bullshit over facts because human beings, multiple studies have shown, prefer bullshit. The very science and technology that brought us cures also encouraged

DIY theorizing. Oceans of digital data only helped us dispense with expertise in favor of our own suppositions and rumor. We are all pseudoscientists, cherry-picking through the new body of knowledge to add supposed credence to old theories about "lizard people" and Bigfoot. Ours is the era of the rise of the citizen expert—the clue hunter, the QAnon "digger" following the trail of crumbs to truth—on the World Wide Web.

The virus arrived at a particular moment in human history when medical advances had dragged us out of the nasty brutishness that defined existence for most of our ancestors. As we've seen, science practically doubled American lifespans in one century. And yet we cannot relinquish the primordial instincts that predispose us to seek a hidden hand behind misfortune and the miracles and magical spells to keep it at bay. The fact that we do live in such a scientific world—buried in a blizzard of data points and facts and the cacophony of beeping updates—enhances the embroidering tendency of our conspiratorial hive mind.

The human brain, researchers are starting to understand, is hard-wired to seek out and prefer conspiracy theories. Resistance is not exactly futile, but it takes sustained vigilance. Even the best-trained scientists are not immune to the urge, as the retired government scientist proved to me on that June night.

The virus is the darkest of all our atomic-era cultural tropes: isolated, in lockdown, living virtual reality, suspicious of our neighbors' very breath, this dystopia was long predicted by science fiction. Covid belongs to Cold War movies like *The Blob* or *Invasion of the Body Snatchers*. Evil geniuses inside labs, working for "lizard people" overlords, release a contagion that turns out to eat brains. Americans have been waiting a long time to see what is really inside Area 51; or Roswell, New

Mexico; or the bioweapons labs over in Fort Detrick, Maryland; or that strange, faraway place called Wuhan.

Now we know.

Besides the human brain's instinct for conspiracy, Covid theories seized the imaginations of so many Americans for another reason. Since the Cold War, science has been implicated in nefarious secrets. Scientists, after all, created the atom bomb, seeding generations to come with an inescapable undertow of terror. After the first weapon of mass destruction, government scientists applied their attention to ever more veiled and heinous activities, from mind control and germ warfare to designing a system of total surveillance via cell phones and the World Wide Web.

Anyone paying the least amount of attention to popular culture or the actual news over the last half-century understands that the US government's storehouse of terrible secrets is vast and growing. The vault is filled with assassinations, poisons, weapons, plots. While it is off-limits to the average citizen, more than five million Americans have security clearances, dwarfing the shrinking number of journalists by orders of magnitude. The national security state metastasized after 9/11 with the Patriot Act. Edward Snowden's revelations revealed just how much the watchers knew or could know.

The fact that the baby boom generation grew up with the metastasization of the national security state has everything to do with the "suspicious minds" of the QAnon crowd, millions of people who coalesced around a bizarre theory that Donald Trump was secretly fighting a global pedophilic elite. Q, after all, presented itself as a mole inside that classified world, perched at the pinnacle of secrets, the Q classification.

Science helped build whatever is inside the locked vault of secrets, and that partly explains why so many Americans don't trust the good science that has healed so many and made life more bearable.

For the older generation, the mysterious virus emerged like a plot point in a Stephen King novel. For the younger crowd, it was just the video game zombie plague. The virus and the novel vaccine that would prevent it, accompanied by scary-sounding phrases like "synthetic genetics," were always destined to become strands in the evolving genome of American paranoia.

GIVE ME LIBERTY

The earliest Covid conspiracy theories were mainstreamed as patriotism. They were broadcast on Fox News and bellowed out from inside the White House. Coronavirus is just like the flu. Anyone who says otherwise wants to crash the stock market and destroy America.

The "flu is just as bad" theory prevailed throughout the first few months of the Covid outbreak. It filled the info vacuum long before hard data was widely available on the virus. Since the early data was contradictory, it was easy to spread controversial analyses, such as a Santa Clara study that underestimated the potential death rate of the virus. Commentary from doubting MDs like Dr. Drew Pinsky made its way into the public consciousness, and, in many cases, never left it—until, one by one, someone's dad or grandma died.

If one believed Covid was no worse than the flu, and if one already distrusted liberals and Democrats and elites and their allied scientists, it was easy to take the next step, to hoax and then to conspiracy. From Fox to right-wing talk radio and social media, the hoax theory was one of the most widespread and enduring.

In the early days of the pandemic, in January and February and March 2020—even in April, when New York City was digging trenches for corpses—the word "hoax" caromed all day across tens of millions of screens tuned to Fox News, while Sean Hannity and Tucker Carlson lambasted Democrats and liberal scientists as alarmists or, worse, liars who were trying to sow panic and destroy Donald Trump's chances of reelection.

Another conservative talking point that took root was that the reported death count from the coronavirus was deceptively inflated. Republicans who wouldn't be caught out in a QAnon hat or at a Trump rally agreed that hospitals were probably getting paid more for Covid deaths. These ideas became bedrock, some of the most widely believed due to their proliferation on media such as Fox News and *The Joe Rogan Experience*, and by President Trump.

The political hoax theory may prove to have caused more American deaths than any single other erroneous belief. It persists on the internet and social media today, long after Fox stopped spreading it. BrandNewTube.com, a YouTube copycat website filled with Covid conspiracy theory videos, has attracted millions of followers. The top two content creators on the site have a combined two million–plus video views. "Dr." (we cannot substantiate the basis for the title) Vernon Coleman is one of the site's most popular Covid conspiracists. Millions listen to him explain how the virus is a hoax to advance an amorphous "elite agenda."

The stream of the pandemic infodemic flowed naturally down to its level, the swamp of politically motivated conspiracy theories on the right. The public health lockdown was only the latest and most egregious strategy employed to advance the liberal elite agenda to crush American liberty, including the right to own guns and private property. No one on the right contradicted this. Libertarian donors like the Koch Foundation got behind the anti-lockdown movement, pouring money and organization into online calls for drive-by rallies at state capitals. Armed men in military regalia who had descended on Richmond, Virginia, in January, just before the pandemic to protest a small change in gun laws, now looked quaint next to the horde that invaded the interior of the capitol building in Lansing, Michigan, in a dry run for the January 6, 2021, insurrection.

Time spent indoors in the early spring: look, it's just a *pause*. Make it fun, do some whittling and watercolors, bake bread, rearrange a hoard of toilet paper rolls, buy gold . . . It's keeping us all safe. On the other hand, if you believed that your office or service job site was shuttered and you were being locked in because of some fake epidemic, every day that went by made you a little bit angrier, or increasingly furious if you tuned in to the conspiracy channels.

One of the most consequential streams of pandemic misinformation was not originally the fault of the Trump administration: not masking. The CDC and the WHO and other experts initially told the public not to worry about masking up. There was a genuine shortage of PPE for medics, and also a group of experts who held sway in communications at the beginning of the pandemic believed that masks would make people complacent about the virus or overconfident, and not do the other things they needed to do, like washing their hands, not touching their faces, and staying away from each other.

By the time the WHO and the CDC changed their mask guidance, it was too late. The technology of misinformation and the politicization of the virus was already baked into the response. The president refused to wear one, and so did his toadies. Masks put a bull's-eye on the members of the elite and their comrades and enablers.

THE KUNG FLU

The first conspiracy theories revolved around the Chinese government and its cover-up. Some of these theories have proven to be somewhat true.

The local authorities in Wuhan, terrified of alarming the public and the Communist Party leadership, initially stifled information. In the spring, Dr. Ai Fen, the director of the emergency department of Wuhan Central Hospital, shared a harrowing personal account of terror and silencing in China's version of *People* magazine. When citizens tried to share her interview on WeChat, Chinese authorities blocked the posts and yanked the original article off the internet. To avoid the censors, people translated Dr. Ai's words into Morse code, emoji, and fictional languages like Sindarin from *The Lord of the Rings*. The account survived and has since been published in English.

As her department filled with patients suffering from a highly contagious strange pneumonia that seemed to affect multiple organ systems, Dr. Ai suspected SARS. She warned her colleagues in an email. Dr. Li Wenliang, a Wuhan ophthalmologist who would later become famous for both blowing the whistle on the dangers of the virus and dying of it, was among the first to share Dr. Ai's message on a WeChat group. Within hours, Dr. Ai received a notice from the city's Health Protection Committee stating that "information on the pneumonia of unknown cause should not be released, to avoid causing panic among the public; if panic was caused by information leaking out there would be an investigation." The next morning, she was called in for a disciplinary review, and told not to tell anyone about the epidemic, including her husband.

"I was utterly stunned," Dr. Ai said. "I had not been criticized for not working hard, but made to feel that what I'd done had ruined Wuhan's prospects and its future."

She stopped talking about it. Throughout the month of January 2020, Dr. Ai watched coughing patients infect her hospital's emergency room and turn critical, and then watched doctors and nurses succumb. She did what she could to protect herself and her staff. She stopped going home. She communicated with her family by video. "My sister helped take care of my children at home," she said. "My youngest child didn't recognize me."

Early on, Dr. Ai understood—and so did her colleagues—that this SARS-like virus was far more contagious than the SARS virus that they knew from the past. They could look at each other falling sick and see that human-to-human transmission was rampant. But Dr. Ai's superiors in the hospital had told her to shut up. It would be weeks before the WHO and the rest of the world acknowledged Covid human-to-human transmission as fact—and another several months before doctors understood that it could be transmitted via air. Precious time was lost protecting China's image.

Lancet editor Richard Horton published one letter he received from an unnamed doctor inside the Chinese medical system pleading for help and asking the outside world to demand transparency. "The Chinese government owes the world a more detailed explanation of what took place in Wuhan," Horton wrote. "I don't mind what we call it—an international inquiry, a fact-finding mission, truth and reconciliation. I don't seek blame. I don't want punishment. I simply want to know what happened. Something happened. We need to know so that we have the best chance of preventing it from happening again."

Conspiracy theories, like nature, thrive in information and knowledge vacuums. They "go viral" in cell cultures of distrust. The Wuhan infodemic swirls with dubious factoids. In early January 2020, as videos of people collapsing on the streets of Wuhan—some real, some fake, who knew?—flooded the internet, a rumor flourished that the death rate matched that of smallpox.

Conspiracy theorists popped up proposing that the virus was a Chinese population control scheme. The "Kung Flu" theory gained traction as rumors leaked out about the mortality of older people. That theory streamed into the grander, global population-control notion I heard about last summer: Bill Gates and the Gates Foundation were spreading the virus as a means to control the exploding world population. Gates personifies the malign "global cabal" theories that fired up Trump's anti-elite "base." Many of these conspiracy theorists also point to a 2015 coronavirus patented by the United Kingdom's Pirbright Institute as evidence that it was a planned pandemic with the goal of lowering the population.

THE LAB-LEAK HYPOTHESIS

The biggest mystery about the virus has to do with its origins.

Did it come out of a bat cave in remote China?

Or did it sneak out of a big-city lab?

The absence of an answer to those questions has invited both amateur and professional theorizing. President Trump, who rarely saw a conspiracy theory he didn't like, proclaimed the lab-leak hypothesis from the White House, during one of his last regular press briefings on the pandemic, on April 30.

A reporter teed him up with a question about whether he had seen evidence that would lead him to conclude with a "high degree of confidence that the Wuhan Institute of Virology was the origin of this virus."

Trump said yes, and added: "The World Health Organization should be ashamed of themselves, because they're like the public relations agency for China. . . . They shouldn't be making excuses when people make horrible mistakes, especially mistakes that are causing hundreds of thousands of people around the world to die."

There are indeed some strange things going on in laboratories all over the world. Real "humanized mice," for example, are the new petri dishes of virology. Developed in the 1980s and refined upon over the years, the humanized mouse is one that has been "xenotransplanted" with human cells or engineered to express human gene products. Genomic breeders churn out on an industrial scale these "chimerics"—cute, white, and fuzzy, with humanlike immune systems. They are so integral to research into Covid that there's a shortage of them in 2021.

Among the strangest of the real *Stranger Things* in infectious disease labs are those that are called "gain of function" experiments. For the last two decades, with the exception of a brief moratorium during the Obama years, researchers have been manipulating animal viruses to make them contagious to humans. The rationale is that if scientists can leap ahead of natural evolution by creating these viruses, they can then also create medicines or techniques to protect humanity from them when they occur naturally.

Hundreds of such experiments have been underway in the

United States and around the world. After 9/11, Dr. Fauci was the lead scientist and director of a US government bioweapons defense program that, among other things, paid scientists to experiment with contagious germs that we are unlikely to encounter unless there is a bioweapons war. The total annual spending on post-9/11 biowarfare defense has been in the hundreds of millions. Some of that money reportedly went to financing gain-of-function experiments in the Wuhan Institute of Virology labs via the Defense Threat Reduction Agency.

In the year before the pandemic, US diplomats based in China were deeply concerned about biosecurity at the Wuhan Institute of Virology, China's first BSL-4 (the highest biosafety level) lab. (At least eleven BSL-4 facilities are currently operating in the United States, according to *New York* magazine.) They cabled Washington with warnings about inexperienced technicians. At some point, US teams may have been dispatched to check it out. The known trail on that story ends there.

The bat virus with the most similar genetic sequence to the coronavirus that causes Covid—discovered to date—existed in nature some one thousand miles from Wuhan, inside a cave where a small group of six miners had become ill, and three had died, of a mysterious pneumonia after shoveling heaps of bat guano. The Chinese released the genome in a timely fashion, proving the virus is closely related to that bat virus. But they refused for a full year to let international teams inspect the Wuhan Institute of Virology.

Shi Zhengli—a prominent Chinese scientist with a long list of official titles: PhD, researcher, director of the Emerging Infectious Diseases Research Center at the Wuhan Institute of Virology, editor in chief of *Virologica Sinica*—went on seven expeditions to the miner's cave and brought the virus that killed them back to her lab at the Wuhan Institute.

It is unclear how or whether she or her researchers experimented on that virus—which was believed to be not highly transmissible among humans—in gain-of-function experiments. Shi has said that her first concern when she learned of the new coronavirus stalking her city was that it might have come from her lab. She has said she immediately checked her papers and found no evidence of the specifically Covid-causing virus in the lab.

The Wuhan Institute of Virology had the world's largest collection of bat viruses in the world. The lab deleted a database of some twenty thousand bat viruses from its website after the pandemic started, citing "national security" reasons. Shi has heaped scorn on lab-leak theorists, telling them to shut their "stinking mouths."

If you've heard any of these curious things before, chances are you first found out about them from one of the myriad online conspiracy theory threads. Very few reputable scientists have spoken out, in a kind of professional circling of the wagons. Those who have, have been criticized. One defender—a Columbia researcher named Angela Rasmussen—even compared the lab-leak theorists to the author of a racist book, *The Turner Diaries*.

The Chinese government has a woeful track record on transparency in pandemic situations. During the deadly 2003 SARS epidemic, officials secretly wheeled sick people out of hospitals before a WHO team entered. They have been censorious on the origins of the Covid virus and forced their own scientists and medics to toe the official line involving a wild animal market.

Some scientists were considering the lab-leak hypothesis from the beginning of the pandemic, but their questions were hijacked by people like Steve Bannon and the rest of the Trumpian Sinophobes. Bannon promoted a dubious story about the virus as a bioweapon. In the early days of Covid, both Trump and Russian state media played up the Chinese lab-leak theory. It was discussed on some widely watched media like *The Joe Rogan Experience*. Banned fascist *Infowars* broadcaster Alex Jones has never stopped airing it. Neither has Reddit.

Since the anti-science, anti-China Trumpists were the first to ring the lab-leak alarm bells, while calling the virus "the China flu" in a racist-nationalist snub, it was easily dismissed. The science community circled the wagons, too. Mainstream media mostly debunked it. But a *New York* magazine article by the novelist and DIY Cold War conspiracy hunter Nicholson Baker—published after Biden won the presidential election—reignited discussion in mainstream media.

In spring 2020, the WHO convened the Independent Panel for Pandemic Preparedness and Response, chaired by the former prime minister of New Zealand, Helen Clark, and the former president of Liberia, Ellen Johnson Sirleaf. The final report of the panel is expected later this year. The British medical journal *Lancet* also established its COVID-19 Commission in July 2020, led by US economist Jeffrey Sachs. It has released an interim statement concluding that SARS-CoV-2 is "a naturally occurring virus, rather than the result of laboratory creation and release."

China finally allowed a WHO team into Wuhan in January 2021. In February, it announced its belief that the virus passed through some as-yet-unknown wild animal into a human—although it averred that the lab-leak theory cannot be ruled out. The WHO's team final report may shed light, but the pro-verbial crime scene has surely been wiped.

Or not.

A year since the virus appeared in Wuhan, and tens of thousands of studies later, science has not identified how the virus mutated from bat to human. (For the record, we also do not know the origin and virulence path of SARS or MERS either.) Once the anti-China, chest-thumping conspiracy theorists of the Trump administration left the world stage, more reputable scientists have stepped up to suggest that the true link between human and bat was not an animal but a lab accident.

Stanford microbiologist Dr. David Relman explained in an interview with me why the hypothesis is reasonable, and why it's hard for scientists to talk about it. "I know that scientists make mistakes and are hesitant to tell the world about them," he said. "If there had been a laboratory accident, think about what the consequences might be. If there were evidence that a benign accident, let's say [by the] Wuhan Institute of Virology, led to this world pandemic and millions of deaths, every one of my colleagues and peers [in] science knows this could have huge, grave consequences for how we view the conduct of sci-ence in laboratories working on infectious agents. It has huge consequences for how we fund science, for oversight, for how decisions are made about what we're going to do and not do."

When Dr. Relman and I spoke, the WHO's investigative team in China had just announced that they were quite sure Covid had jumped from bat to human by an as-yet-unidentified animal. A lab leak was the least likely option, according to the team.

COLD WAR SCIENCE

A sub-theory of the Chinese lab-leak theory is that the virus originated as an experimental bioweapon in either China or the United States, and was either intentionally leaked into the public, stolen, or released in an accidental fashion similar to the original hypothesis.

The story of US government experiments and bioweapons is mostly buried in top secret files and redacted documents. The United States started its bioweapons project during World War II, in response to German and Japanese bioweapons research. Thousands of scientists were recruited to work at Fort Detrick, Maryland. The fascist governments in Germany and Japan were running horrendous bioweapons experiments on captive humans—free of any moral or ethical restrictions. After the war, the Central Intelligence Agency (CIA) rescued some of these mad scientists from war crimes charges, and brought them over to the United States to share their knowledge at Fort Detrick.

During the Cold War, Fort Detrick's projects ramped up. The United States used at least one of the inventions conceived of at Fort Detrick—feathers or insects laden with bacteria—to attack North Korea. Some of the details in Stephen Kinzer's book about the mastermind behind the great leaps forward in this realm, the CIA's "poisoner in chief" Dr. Sidney Gottlieb, are almost too horrifying to read.

American bioweapons research waned after various US-USSR détentes, and when the Berlin Wall fell the budget for it diminished even further. But 9/11 prompted a new blast of funding, and hundreds of millions poured into research.

All of it classified.

Who can blame anyone for weaving horror stories from these facts?

The full history of American bioweapons research continues to tantalize researchers and stoke paranoia more than anything else the US government has done. Novelist Nicholson Baker made a project of FOIAing the US government to try to get at the truth of the projects, and wrote about his trip down this rabbit hole in a book, *Baseless*. Baker concluded that enough unclassified information exists to support a startling theory— that US germ warrior experiments on weaponizing a plant disease aimed at wheat to starve the Soviet Army got loose in the homeland in the 1950s and caused crop failures in fourteen US states. Baker also seems to favor the theory that another mad government experiment on weaponizing ticks loosed Lyme disease on America.

The Cold War and germ warfare experiments were not the end of this morally dubious research. Gain-of-function operations sound like dystopic fantasy fiction. For experiments on animal respiratory viruses, researchers have developed cell cultures out of human windpipes. The cultures grow cilia and mucus, just like the human breathing organ. The gain-of-function experiments grow animal viruses in the lung-like cultures, over and over, until the pathogens evolve to target human lung cells.

Then the newly infectious creations are stored in freezers, supposedly to be used for therapeutic and vaccine experiments to prevent a natural pandemic—or to defend against a foreign biological attack.

Many scientists have questioned the wisdom of these operations. Gain-of-function viruses are not bioweapons, but their funding has sometimes intermingled with money for defense. The US government's various agencies—the Pentagon, HHS, the NIH (including work overseen by Dr. Fauci)—have supported the research. In theory, the studies might lead to preemptive vaccines and cures—in case the viruses were ever to become human contagions.

The fact that Dr. Fauci oversaw top secret bioweapon and gain-of-function research has provoked many memes and theories among conspiracy-minded anti-vaxxers. It is further proof for them that the nation's favorite doctor is not only lying about the virus and the vaccine, he is covering up for more powerful puppet masters.

In October 2019, top US national security officials and private security groups participated in Event 201—a pandemic "tabletop exercise" hosted by the Johns Hopkins Center for Health Security. These exercises are like kaffeeklatsches for the policy and science set. Foundations host them regularly to analyze preparedness, from hypothetical nuclear attacks to asteroid hits. VIPs and Nobel prizewinners fly in from distant shores to rub elbows imagining how they could handle the worst.

Event 201 participants included representatives from the World Economic Forum and the Bill & Melinda Gates Foundation.

Half a year after the pandemic started, a group of Italian researchers reported that they believed the coronavirus was circulating in Italy already in September 2019. Their new timeline hasn't been confirmed by other scientists. But it gave the Event 201 deep state theory new credence. Perhaps the gathering was some kind of real-life emergency response.

Online suspicions about this event prompted Johns Hopkins to release a public denial. The exercise was not looking at anything real. "Recently, the Center for Health Security has received questions about whether that pandemic exercise predicted the current novel coronavirus outbreak in China," the press release stated. "To be clear, the Center for Health Security and partners did not make a prediction during our tabletop exercise. For the scenario, we modeled a fictional coronavirus pandemic, but we explicitly stated that it was not a prediction. Instead, the exercise served to highlight preparedness and response challenges that would likely arise in a very severe pandemic. We are not now predicting that the nCoV-2019 outbreak will kill 65 million people. Although our tabletop exercise included a mock novel coronavirus, the inputs we used for modeling the potential impact of that fictional virus are not similar to nCoV-2019."

The Chinese have their own deep state theory, absolving them of blame. In their theory, the zoonotic virus was deliberately enhanced in a gain-of-function experiment inside US bioweapons labs at Fort Detrick. Chinese state media increased its attention to this theory as the Pfizer vaccine was found to be more efficacious than China's Sinovac antibody vaccine in early 2021.

A third version of the bioweapons theory—favored by Reddit conspiracy buffs—is that Chinese nationals, working in US labs, stole the American lab-enhanced coronavirus variant and brought it back to China, where it was accidentally or deliberately leaked.

This theory relies on factual reports of US charges against Chinese lab workers at Harvard bio labs—arrests that had nothing to do with coronavirus research.

Farther down the rabbit hole, on 4chan, posters have proposed that Covid was deliberately spread through vapes.

THE GREAT RESET

The tabletop pandemic exercise months before the real one is just one example. We could write an entire multi-tome encyclopedia about the good intentions gone awry of the Davos set. Had we but world enough and time . . . But we don't.

Fact: you can hate Microsoft Word's glitches and bugs and still acknowledge the fact that Bill Gates's philanthropy is responsible for saving the lives of millions of children in developing countries thanks to its vaccination programs.

Conspiracy: in his home country, 28 percent of Americans and 44 percent of Republicans in May 2020 believed that Bill Gates wanted to use vaccines to implant microchips in people. (This means that if you live next door to a Republican family, one of every two members of the household might, if you got close enough, tell you that.)

Global philanthropic organizations like the Bill & Melinda Gates Foundation have taken frontline roles in vaccinating children for diarrheal disease and working in AIDS prevention and searching for a cure for that disease, vaccinating the world's poor against multiple diseases and saving millions of lives. Many vaccine programs, though, have provoked rumor and distrust, here and abroad. Some Africans and Asians have suspected the vaccines are forced sterilization programs, and there's been violent resistance, including murders of public health workers. Even in the United States, one can find claims that the AIDS epidemic is a man-made government plot.

Whether or not they pay the fantasies of the rabble any heed, the philanthropists and their friends in the Davos world tend to favor language that is easily manipulated into "world domination" theories by suspicious minds. During the pandemic, "the Great Reset" conspiracy has seized the imaginations of untold millions.

The Great Reset is the title of a book by an economist named Richard Florida, and corporate sustainability types now like to throw it around to give their projects a futuristic spark. But in the summer of 2020, the World Economic Forum and the British royal family's Sustainable Markets Initiative announced a new goal proposing to redirect investments to sustainable industry. They hashtagged it #thegreatreset and put out a video with polar bears and ice floes and music. But conspiracists had seen too many dying polar bears to be fooled by the title. There it was—everything they suspected about the elite plot against the masses.

They weren't even trying to hide it!

The *Guardian* reported what happened next: "Weeks after the WEF's announcement, Justin Haskins, the editorial director of the libertarian thinktank, the Heartland Institute, sounded klaxons about the great reset on Fox Business, Fox News and Glenn Beck's network, TheBlaze. 'The rough outline of the plan is clear,' he said. 'Completely destroy the global capitalist economy and reform the western world.'"

In October 2020, conservative Catholic archbishop Carlo Maria Vigano wrote an open letter to President Trump: "A global plan called the Great Reset is underway. Its architect is a global élite that wants to subdue all of humanity, imposing coercive measures with which to drastically limit individual freedoms and those of entire populations. In several nations this plan has already been approved and financed; in others it is still in an early stage. Behind the world leaders who are the accomplices and executors of this infernal project, there are unscrupulous characters who finance the World Economic Forum and Event 201, promoting their agenda."

The "infernal project" finally caught fire after Joe Biden's presidential victory, when searches for the term surged online.

"The Great Reset" theory is the broadest version of the grand unifying theory I first noticed in the Midwest. Its villainology encompasses almost all the usual suspects under a single umbrella belief system, including, but not limited to, Bill Gates and the Gates Foundation, Dr. Anthony Fauci, China, Joe Biden and the Clintons, George Soros, the CIA, Jews, Muslims, the medical industry, corporate media, and the wireless data industry.

BLEACH, FISH TANK CLEANER, 5G FEVER

Science can tell us a lot about the virus. Thanks to good science, and the nature of the pandemic's infodemic, more humans know more about this virus than humans have ever known about any virus before. Researchers accomplished a secular miracle creating six efficacious vaccines within a year.

But science was never a match for the DIY medical world.

On March 22, 2020, Wanda and Gary Lenius, a Phoenix, Arizona, couple in their late sixties, feeling a bit ill, decided to ward off what they thought were cases of Covid by each adding a teaspoon of a fish tank cleaner containing chloroquine phosphate into some soda and drinking it. Within minutes, Wanda was vomiting and Gary was having respiratory problems. They called an ambulance. Gary died. Wanda survived after a stint in intensive care.

What were they thinking? They had decided to test President Trump's advice about a miracle cure for Covid, called hydroxychloroquine. "We saw [Trump's] press conference," Wanda said later. "It was on a lot, actually. Trump kept saying it was pretty much a cure."

The bark extracts of the cinchona tree were used in Peru to treat malaria and babesiosis as long as four hundred years ago. Medical science isolated the reason why it worked—quinine—two hundred years later. Chloroquine has been used to treat malaria since the 1930s, but it has terrible side effects. A variation of the drug, hydroxychloroquine, with fewer side effects, is sold under the brand name Plaquenil for malaria and autoimmune diseases. In its fish bowl cleaner version, the chemical saves fish, but is toxic to humans.

The day after the hospital announced that Gary Lenius had died, across the country in New York, authorities shut down a Russian émigré doctor whose claims he had kept more than five hundred Covid-symptomatic patients out of the hospital by using hydroxychloroquine had attracted President Trump's attention.

By afternoon, Dr. Vladimir Zelenko was up and running again. The White House had intervened with the state officials. Dr. Zelenko was directing what the *Forward* called at the time "perhaps the world's most extensive, unsanctioned medical experiment related to coronavirus—the use of the anti-malaria drug hydroxychloroquine to treat Covid-19."

Like the Silicon Valley engineer who got Trump's attention with a tweet and won an $86 million ventilator contract, Dr. Zelenko had caught the president's fancy via the usual ad hoc avenues—social media and the right-wing echo chamber. Trump was soon touting the drug as a "game changer" as Sean Hannity promoted Dr. Zelenko's claims on his TV and radio shows, incoming White House chief of staff Mark Meadows called Zelenko personally, and Rudy Giuliani hailed Zelenko on a podcast for "thinking of solutions, just like the president."

Eventually the scientific method prevailed over the DIY self-medicators. Dr. Fauci called evidence of the drug's efficacy "anecdotal." It was known to be dangerous for the severely ill. On the morning of March 24, New York banned the off-label use of the drug outside state-sanctioned clinical trials.

Game on!

That afternoon, Vice President Mike Pence announced that the FDA was approving off-label use of the drug "right now." Pence announced: "Doctors can now prescribe chloroquine for that off-label purpose of dealing with the symptoms of corona-virus."

Trump soon strong-armed his FDA into emergency approval of its use. On April 5, the FDA commissioner, Dr. Stephen Hahn, contacted Dr. Zelenko and asked if he had "time for a quick call." When he got Dr. Zelenko on the phone, Dr. Hahn asked how he could be of help. He then told the doctor to reach out to FEMA to obtain hydroxychloroquine from the Strategic National Stockpile. Dr. Hahn offered, "I'll send you the contact."

(It's important to remember here that the Trump adminis-tration never bothered to activate the FEMA stockpile for PPE, nor felt any urgency to force the FDA to approve non-CDC Covid tests when mass testing might have got the pandemic under control. Of course not: he liked the numbers low.)

In Trumpworld, Gary Lenius was a minor martyr fallen along the road to rapid economic reopening.

In May, Trump announced he was "taking the hydroxy."

The president liked to dispense his own medical knowledge, because, after all, he was a kind of genius.

On April 23, at one of the Mad Hatter's tea party White House nightly pandemic news briefings that put a coda to those horrible early days for Americans, Trump had some new good news. William Bryan, the undersecretary for science and technology at the Department of Homeland Security, briefly presented a study that found sun exposure and cleaning agents like bleach can kill the virus when it lingers on surfaces.

Trump then took the podium and riffed on the salubrious effects of disinfectants and UV light on the human body. The "drink bleach" moment became one of the enduring memes of his presidency. To be fair, the president did not actually tell people to drink bleach. He just mused on the possibility that it could be injected into the lungs.

Coming a month after the fish bowl cleaner death, Trump's remarks led bleach companies and state agencies to issue warnings about ingesting disinfectants. Lysol issued a statement that "under no circumstance" should its products be used in the human body. Clorox posted: "Bleach and other disinfectants are not suitable for consumption or injection under any circumstances." (The notice remains on the company website.)

Hilarity and horror. It was a meme. Trump wants doctors to inject you with bleach. The White House was black comedy, a modern Weimar cabaret. Three days later, Trump threw in the towel on the Covid briefings, labeling them "not worth the time and effort."

Conspiracy theorists in the Trump camp always thought Trump was being ridiculed unfairly. Like Michael Caputo, the cracked communications director at the CDC, millions of people were on the verge of losing their minds over "deep state public health" and its nefarious agenda.

There was more, of course. Many not only distrusted the deep state, but dispensed with faith in the existence of microbes altogether. These people—an international community, actually—believe 5G networks being erected in many countries are the true source of the new sickness. Since spring 2020, anti-5G individuals have been attacking cell tower workers around the world to protect themselves and their communities from the Covid-inducing wireless rays. The theory gained a lot of traction in the United Kingdom before the QAnon conspiracy boards picked it up. Actor Woody Harrelson is among the high-profile 5G conspiracy adherents. So, possibly, was the Tennessee RV bomber.

This was the state of the world in which the utterly new vaccines would be dropped.

THE ANTI-VAXXERS

Vaccine hesitancy is nearly as old as vaccines. As the cowpox vaccine entered wider use, circa 1800, cartoonist James Gillray depicted people who had received the vaccine taking on bovine attributes, with snouts, tails, and floppy cow ears. The first organized anti-vaccine league formed in Britain in the 1850s as the government tried to make smallpox vaccination mandatory. Vaccine side effects and vaccine errors during the early twentieth century eroded trust as high-profile errors like the polio vaccine accidents joined a list of terrifying risks that tended to overshadow the safety records and vast successes of most vaccine campaigns. As the US government increased the number of vaccines that parents must give their children (up to fifteen now), some parents resisted.

The modern anti-vaccine movement coalesced in 1998, after a British doctor, Andrew Wakefield (who subsequently lost his medical license), published a study claiming a link between autism and the vaccine for measles, mumps, and rubella. The study was widely shared. And it was false. The publisher, the *Lancet*, retracted it twelve years later, but not before immunization rates in some countries dropped sharply.

Wakefield was a gastroenterologist at the Royal Free Hospital in London when he ran a study on twelve children. Once the study was published, Wakefield gave a news conference and made a blanket statement opposing the use of the vaccine. Wakefield became a hero to parents of autistic kids and traveled the United States, addressed autism conferences, and appeared on *60 Minutes*.

His study remains the founding document for a vast community of believers twenty years later. It makes no difference how many times he or it has been debunked. Seth Mnookin, a science writer and professor at the Massachusetts Institute of Technology, has written that the study "wasn't built on a house of cards" because "there weren't any cards to begin with." An investigative journalist discovered that Wakefield was on the payroll of lawyers who planned to sue the vaccine makers.

The anti-vaccination movement crosses socioeconomic and educational lines. Pediatrician and infectious diseases expert Dr. Paul Offit, co-inventor of the rotavirus disease vaccine that has saved millions of children in the developing world, blames what he calls the "devaluing" of expertise, DIY culture, and the internet for the proliferation of distrust.

When anti-vaxxers kicked off a measles outbreak a few years ago that spread to twenty-five states, Dr. Offit looked into the communities behind it. "If you look at the demographics, those were people who were college-educated, I'll say graduate-school-educated, Caucasian, suburban, who had jobs in which they exercise some level of control," he said. "Who believe that they could look on the internet and know just as much as anybody who gave them advice. It's this sort of 'I can know as much as anybody else because I have access to information that I can find on the internet.' And so it's a devaluing of expertise and a devaluing of experience.

"I don't think those same people do that with regard to say, fixing their car," Dr. Offit continued. "You know, if they're going to have a gallbladder operation, I don't think they go to the surgeon and say, 'I've been looking on the internet. I'd really prefer this posterior, rather than the anterior approach.' I don't think they do that. But I think with regard to vaccines or this sort of thing, they think they can do it."

After the logistical challenges of distribution, one of the greatest impediments to getting Covid shots into enough arms to reach 80 percent, the threshold of herd or community immunity, may be the anti-vaxxer movement.

The anti-vaxxer community was activated before the emergency use approval. They spread the lie that Dr. Elisa Granato, one of the first participants in an early Oxford-AstraZeneca vaccine trial, had died. Dr. Granato tweeted out that she was "very much alive" and "having a cup of tea."

In the United States, anti-vaccination groups published Facebook pages and YouTube videos with large followings long before Covid. Anti-vaccine activist Del Bigtree lost his YouTube channel after he minimized the coronavirus pandemic, telling viewers to intentionally expose themselves to Covid. Facebook took down his Informed Consent Action Network page, which had more than 360,000 followers, but not before it shared more than five hundred videos attracting more than thirty million views.

Researchers studied one hundred million people who had expressed views about vaccination and found that while the anti-vaccination community is relatively small, its message is "robust and resilient" because its conspiracy theories are more widely shared than the more boring truths about risk and reward. The researchers concluded that anti-vaccination views will dominate within a decade.

Foot soldiers in the vaccine and pandemic preparedness community have been fighting back for years. Heidi Larson heads a British effort, the Vaccine Confidence Project, and had just finished a book about her adventures pushing vaccines against rumor and lies when the pandemic broke out. It's called *Stuck*. Her conclusion about vaccine hesitation: "We don't have a misinformation problem. We have a trust problem."

The anti-vaccine community already had a big head start when the first Covid vaccines were approved for emergency use in the United Kingdom and then in the United States. Within hours of the announcement that the Pfizer vaccine had been approved for use in the United Kingdom, the internet was flooded with social media posts urging people not to accept it. The word "thalidomide" soon began trending on Twitter.

NATURE'S WAY

The Covid vaccine conspiracies run the gamut from the outlandish (the vaccines cause HIV, they contain tracking microchips) to the politically targeted (they are made with aborted fetal tissue). One of the most common and effective misconceptions about the Pfizer and Moderna vaccines is that they affect a person at the very core, at the DNA level. The mere mention of "messenger RNA" in the vaccine sends a flicker of unease through millions of GMO-wary consumers.

Online wellness influencers who hawk "natural" cures are also involved. Home-birthers and devotees of vitamins and acupuncture and organic baby food prefer to trust Mother Nature. The tone of the online discussions is always DIY "common sense" versus educated condescension, like this Twitter exchange between Kentucky Republican representative Thomas Massie and former Clinton White House press secretary Joe Lockhart. Massie tweeted: "Which immunity is superior? Vaccines shown to be 70-90% effective at 7-14 days based on a few hundred cases of COVID-19 or Natural Immunity shown to be 99.999% effective at 8 months based on a few million cases." Massie's tweet had racked up almost eight thousand "likes" by the time Lockhart shot at him, "Are you really that dumb or just pretending?"

The "natural way" argument is appealing to a wide variety of interests. It potentially brings together the progressive, organic, wellness yoga crowd and the conservative, mask-free, rugged, social-Darwinian cowboy crowd.

Epidemiologist Jessica Malaty Rivera studies "infodemiology," and she is familiar with the nature-knows-better argument against vaccines. She has a neologism for it: "chemophobia."

"It's a logical fallacy," she said of the nature-knows-better argument. "There's genetic material in literally everything. In the bananas that are in your organic smoothie, in the blueberries that you eat on the fly, everything has chemicals, everything has some sort of genetic material. I think chemophobia is the underlying issue here, that people think chemical is antithetical to nature, but nature is full of chemicals. When they hear mRNA, they think genetic material, genetic material means genetic modification, that means cyborgs, and aliens, and robots. It's just such a leap from the truth."

TRUST AND THE DEEP STATE

The pandemic hit America after a three-year war on expertise, facts, science, and data across all levels of the government. Trump signaled the new era on day one of his administration, when he sent Sean Spicer out to try to persuade Americans that his inauguration crowd was bigger than Obama's, perhaps the largest in American history. Photographs and law enforcement and media estimates of the numbers indicating otherwise were #fakenews.

After that, the Trump administration set about scrubbing data everywhere. It took climate change and pollution data off the Environmental Protection Agency's websites. Government scientists, like people in a house fire, grabbed what they could before the files disappeared.

In midsummer 2020, the Trump regime, emboldened by the success of nearly four years of shoveling facts into the incinerator, quietly pulled off one of its more audacious and egregious data-stifling efforts. The Department of Health and Human Services officially instructed American hospitals to stop feeding numbers of Covid patients to the CDC and instead to hand it over to a small, private Pittsburgh-based firm, TeleTracking, whose majority owner is (but of course) a Trump donor and real estate developer.

At the meeting where this change was announced, one CDC employee reportedly fled the room in tears, saying, "I refuse to do this. I cannot work with people like this. It is so toxic." (One can fill in the eye rolls and laughter over this at the Trump International bar later that evening.)

Trump's HHS also scrubbed the nation's historical Covid data from the CDC's website. A public outcry forced HHS to replace it, but the CDC numbers were no longer updated. Meanwhile, TeleTracking's data was flawed and slow to update, putting the United States at a disadvantage compared with other countries in efforts to track and mitigate outbreaks at their source.

Operating from his perch in the West Wing, Jared Kushner presided over another crony data-collection operation. He put

Silicon Valley pals and eventually the surveillance giant Palantir (owned by a rare pro-Trump Silicon Valley titan, Peter Thiel) in charge of a separate Covid data system. Besides adding another layer of separate requests for information to beleaguered hospitals and agencies, Kushner made policy decisions based on this separate data chain. In March, Kushner contradicted New York governor Andrew Cuomo's pleas for thirty thousand more ventilators, claiming New York State didn't need them. "I'm doing my own projections, and I've gotten a lot smarter about this," Kushner said.

In American society, not just politics, there is a cultural link between real estate scion Jared Kushner doing his own health data projections and "getting a lot smarter about this" and the QAnon crowd doing their digging and knowing better than the journalists and the scientists about just about everything.

The challenges of vaccinating hundreds of millions of Americans subject to this level of arrogance, paranoia, and distrust of authority sounded insurmountable. In April 2020, the Pew Research Center estimated that one in three Americans believe Covid is man-made. And the Pentagon reported that up to a third of some troops were refusing the vaccination. Getting a vaccination into every single man, woman, and child in America requires a compliant society that trusts centralized medical databases. Such a project can't work with a large demographic that will freak out and think that Bill Gates/lizard people/the Chinese have invaded when they see men and women in camo setting up tents down the street to stick them with a serum.

In all this, there is a tiny glimmer of good news.

After four years of anti-science ascendancy in which amateurs and autodidacts controlled all the levers of American government and lies became truth, it may come as a surprise to hear that the foundation of secular, reality-based society has not in fact crumbled. Pew researchers find that the vast majority of Americans—86 percent—are confident that scientists act in the public interest. That includes a subset of 35 percent of Americans who have "a great deal of confidence"—up from 21 percent in 2016. And it hasn't really changed much over the years.

Of course, everyone could be lying about that too.

Maybe only the lizard people respond to surveys these days.

CHAPTER 5

The Land of the Free

Who telleth a tale of unspeaking death?
Who lifteth the veil of what is to come?
Who painteth the shadows that are beneath
The wide-winding caves of the peopled tomb?

—from PERCY BYSSHE SHELLEY's "On Death"

TOMBER AUX OUBLIETTES

The second Moderna shot made me sick—as predicted.

A twenty-four-hour touch of what an alarmed immune system feels like made me all the more grateful for my good fortune in avoiding the real thing, and to be alive at a time when science had devised a 95 percent effective vaccine in record time.

To distract myself from the fever as I tried to sleep, I visualized strands of synthetic messenger RNA floating into my cells to produce the alien spike protein that attracted my warrior T cells. I drifted off envisioning an epic micro-battle underway in my blood, and had a series of weird nightmares. At about 2 a.m., I woke up sweating and disoriented and nauseated, fixated on a grim image from Arthur Allen's book *Vaccine: The Controversial Story of Medicine's Greatest Lifesaver*. In the days of ignorance—not so very long ago—doctors prescribed "hot air baths" for the feverish victims of deadly epidemics of smallpox or yellow fever, clamping them under woolen covers in closed rooms with the windows shut.

Mildly claustrophobic in the best of times, my mind scrabbled to other forms of medical persecution I'd read about. In the American colonies, for example, whether or not to take the Jenner cowpox vaccine was a matter of religious concern—the role of clerics in torture has its own literary genre, of course. Puritans were taught that they interfered with God's will when they altered the outcomes of disease. To expiate that sin, or more likely out of sheer ignorance, medical doctors of the day decreed that the cowpox vaccine would only work after weeks of purging, including ingesting mercury, which besides making people drool and have diarrhea, also loosened their teeth.

"Inoculation meant three weeks of daily vomiting, purges, sweats, fevers," Allen wrote. He includes an account of the suffering inflicted on a twelve-year-old Boston boy before he was inoculated in April 1764. "Sunday we took a powder in the morning that work'd me nine times. . . . Monday morning took two pills which worked me twice. . . . Tuesday took a powder that work'd me ten times. . . . Thursday took a powder that worked me 5 times up and once down. . . . Saturday April 21 took a powder which work'd me 4 times up and one down. Felt very sick in the Morning and did not get up till 10 o'clock. . . . At night took brimstone [sulfur] in Milk for a sore mouth."

John Adams, before he was president of the United States, suffered similarly in preparation for his vaccination. "A long and total abstinence from everything in nature that has any taste, two heavy vomits, one heavy Cathartick, four and twenty mercurial and antinomial pills and three weeks close confinement in house."

To clear my thoughts, I opened my window to let in the winter air and breathed deep. I leaned out and into the pandemic's clean black sky, the starlight so much brighter since the jets stopped flying and we ceased driving and burning so much coal. Silence.

An inkling of what the world might be like without us.

Chilled, I lay back down and wondered: What will the future think of us in this time? Will they recoil in horror as I just did, looking in a fever nightmare at the generations that came before us?

When America reached the half-million-dead mark at the end of February 2021, reports compared the number to our glorious war dead. The pandemic had now killed more Americans than World War I, World War II, and the Vietnam War combined, and it wasn't done with us yet. But the Covid dead had not marched into battle. They had gone off to their jobs as bus drivers and nurses and store clerks, or hugged a grandchild, or been too close to a care worker who arrived at a nursing home via the subway.

The world remembers and celebrates the date of the end of World War I every November 11 on Armistice—now called Veterans—Day. But the last great pandemic, the Spanish flu, which killed fifty million people—including more World War I soldiers than were killed by other men and killing machines—has fallen into a collective memory hole.

Our grandparents and great-grandparents turned away and did not look back. Donald Trump's grandfather's death from the Spanish flu in 1919 changed the fortunes of his family forever. And yet Trump never spoke of it—even while presiding over a great and similar natural disaster. This forgetting wasn't just a Trumpian aberrance. It is a cultural phenomenon. My own doctor in New York remembers how his grandfather never made much of having survived the Spanish flu. The old man remembered watching his sister die of it, but "it was as if it was not unusual, as if it was just something that happened." *Lancet* editor Richard Horton has talked about this forgetting phenomenon. "There was no memory of [the 1918 pandemic] imprinted on our culture. And nobody fully understands why that is. Maybe people just wanted desperately to look forward and not back."

As hard as it is to imagine right now, it's possible that future generations will forget our pandemic as well.

Medical anthropologist Martha Louise Lincoln believes the tendency to look forward—and away from disaster—is an American habit. "Collectively, we obviously wrongly shared a feeling that Americans would be fine," Lincoln said of the early days of the Covid pandemic. "I think that's in part because of the way we're conditioned to remember history.

"We misremember our experiences of war, particularly in a really self-interested way," she continued. "And then when we inevitably compare pandemics to wars, we're cuing Americans to think that it's going to go well for us, even though, of course, our wars don't go that well for us.

"We ultimately end up remembering, even Vietnam—really terrible foreign policy adventures—somehow as stories about the endurance of Americans, the resilience of Americans, when what we really should be remembering is the capacity of Americans to go in unprepared.

"We have a collective cognitive resistance to seeing ourselves as able to lose," Lincoln concluded. "We don't really know or appreciate in our bones what losing feels like. Even though American history is full of painful losses, we don't take them in."

We are very likely to overcome the virus at some point in the not-too-distant future. As hard as it is to imagine right now, the menace that shut down the planet will be brought to heel by vaccines. In years to come, it will still afflict humanity, but as nothing more than "an annoying childhood infection." And there will be an unforeseen benefit, because the pandemic provoked such a proliferation of research into coronaviruses that scientists are even suggesting a vaccine for the common cold (also a coronavirus) is a possibility.

We were very, very lucky—Covid is relatively benign compared with Ebola or MERS. As a species, we will survive this one. It was bad, but it could have been much worse. Sociologist and writer Zeynep Tufekci has called it "a starter pandemic."

It may be that the creation of these new mRNA vaccines means we'll be lucky again the next time. We will not forget; we will heed some of the lessons.

Perhaps our leaders will keep an office for a pandemic preparedness team in a corner of the national security apparatus—and give a scientist the president's cell phone number.

Within weeks of coming into office at the end of the first year of the pandemic, a new president indeed filled the vacant position of White House science adviser—left unfilled by the previous occupant, who didn't like to have that kind of smarty-pants around. The new science adviser is a geneticist, Eric Lander, a man who can read a genome, the coded language that will lead us out of this and future pandemics.

The pandemic might even persuade some of the skeptics and science doubters that it really was science—not God, not President Trump—that saved us. This wasn't a "Great Reset"; Bill Gates didn't inject everyone with 5G trackers. It was just human science, combining with vast, new technological ability paired with artificial intelligence, fighting and winning a battle against an eternal and always-changing foe.

We must try *not* to forget this moment and what it feels like, because the number of pathogens waiting to jump from mammals to us is alarmingly large. Modern human activity has made us more, not less, vulnerable to another pandemic. It is not a matter of if, but when.

A University of Liverpool study published in February 2021 applied artificial intelligence to predict relationships between 411 strains of coronavirus and 876 potential mammalian host species and found at least eleven times more associations between species and coronavirus strains than have been observed to date. They found over forty times more mammal species that can be infected with coronavirus strains than were previously known. The Covid coronavirus could easily recombine with any of them, a fact the researchers deemed an immediate public health threat.

We may in fact be entering a new "era of pandemics," according to a study produced during an "urgent virtual workshop" convened in October 2020 by the United Nations' Intergovernmental Science-Policy Platform on Biodiversity and Ecosystem Services (ISPPBES) to investigate the links between pandemic risk and the degradation of nature.

Due to climate change, intense agriculture, unsustainable trade, misuse of land, and nature-disrupting production and consumption habits, more than five new diseases emerge in people every year, any one of which could potentially spark a pandemic.

The ISPPBES predicted that "future pandemics will emerge more often, spread more rapidly, do more damage to the world economy, and kill more people than COVID-19, unless there is a transformative change in the global approach to dealing with infectious diseases."

The ISPPBES recommended establishing an intergovern-mental panel of pandemic prevention and setting up a global monitoring mechanism that would set international goals and benchmarks to reduce damaging consumption habits and agricultural practices.

THE LAND OF THE FREE

In this book, we have covered the murderous decisions—linked to the celebration of ignorance and greed, MBA ideology, cronyism, and the politicization of the virus—specific to Trump's regime. But, as we have seen, one pandemic failure did not originate with the Trump administration. The CDC and the WHO's initial guidance on not wearing masks, however well intentioned, validated enduring doubt about masks' efficacy even after the experts reversed their position. By then, masks had been politicized by Trump and his allies, and covering one's nose and mouth was like wearing a "Biden for President" T-shirt.

In June 2020, Goldman Sachs, no pal to the proletariat, released a report on mask wearing and the economy, using an algorithm it called the "Effective Lockdown Index" (ELI). Applying the ELI, Goldman's analysts determined that a national mask mandate "could potentially substitute for lockdowns that would otherwise subtract nearly 5% from GDP." But by then it was already too late. No economic analysis could change the dynamic which equated face-mask-wearing with socialist Big Brother totalitarianism, the very opposite of Trump's flavor of American freedom as symbolized by the red MAGA cap.

All those red-blooded, liberty-loving Americans ripping their masks off and fighting with store managers in Target and

Walmart saw themselves as patriots battling an invasive, all-seeing state authority like China.

But as Americans, they have already submitted abjectly to a total intrusion: cryptic mass commercial data harvesting. Billions of bits of their personal data stream minute by minute, click by click, into the great underground sea tapped by private enterprise without anyone's explicit consent. Google, Facebook, and their spawn of apps collect, study, and sell hundreds of thousands of collateral data points on every man, woman, and child in the nation. Facebook's well-known mass-behavioral experiments, the advanced "reality mining" operations of the Massachusetts Institute of Technology's media lab, are just the better known of thousands of projects underway enabled by a system of data collection that we are rarely asked to consent to.

Shoshana Zuboff, in her book *The Age of Surveillance Capitalism*, calls the recipients and manipulators of this collateral behavioral data collectively "Big Other." In theory, Big Other's all-seeing eye could make tracking and controlling a public health crisis easier than ever in human history. The proliferation of health data apps on American smartphones had reached more than one hundred thousand in 2016. But the data collected by those apps is sold to help merchants sell stuff, not to help public health officials. Wearable sensor technologies, smart home technology, and other health-monitoring artificial intelligence in development are all designed in the service of commercial interests.

All that data isn't streaming into doctor's offices, or flowing into a local or national public health database. Few Americans—and certainly not the anti-maskers—would accept such intrusion. But we submit without a fuss to much greater *commercial* privacy intrusions, and we know from Edward

Snowden that the national security state can dip into the data stream any time it wants.

Republicans—the party of unmasking and "liberty"—have consistently supported surveillance capitalism. As recently as 2017, they voted against giving individuals the power to even consent to having their data hoovered up and sold by cable and phone companies for ads and profiling.

"It is eloquent testimony to the health care system's failure to serve the needs of second-modernity individuals that we now access health data and advice from our phones while these pocket computers aggressively access us," Zuboff wrote. She added that the growing habit of online medical searches "has triggered an explosion of rendition and behavioral surplus capture as individuals turn in record numbers to their fitness bands and apps for support and guidance."

The pandemic crisis is a good time to ask: Could some of that surveillance capacity be harnessed to streamline and connect public health efforts, to predict and ease health crises like the pandemic? And even if the industry could create a centralized system for tracking the sick, the exposed, the unvaccinated, would we want it?

Policy makers, Big Tech, electronic privacy advocates, and the public have barely begun to think about how to apply technology in a way that doesn't turn Western societies into China-like authoritarian dystopias. We've not been asked, until now.

Before the pandemic, there was very little interest in harnessing tech to public health. One notable exception was when Big Tech stepped in to save the disastrous 2013 Obamacare rollout on the healthcare.gov website. "Digital health is more new than improved and sorely in need of more significant results rather than facile claims," wrote Vanessa Mason, founder of a public health tech venture fund, in a 2017 plea entitled "Dear Silicon Valley, It Pays to Care About Public Health."

Public health is neither sexy nor lucrative, and Silicon Valley's products are created almost solely by men with two chief aims: to get rich and to get laid. Recall that early incarnations of Siri could find prostitutes and Viagra but not abortion providers. The tech titans came to power applying algorithmic skills toward creating platforms aimed at ever more finely targeted ads and helping math nerds meet girls. Reviewing the movie *The Social Network*, the writer Zadie Smith wrote that everything about Facebook is "reduced to the size of its founder. Poking, because that's what shy boys do to girls they are scared to talk to." Ultimately, she wrote, *The Social Network* wasn't "a cruel portrait of any particular real-world person called 'Mark Zuckerberg.' It's a cruel portrait of us: 500 million sentient people entrapped in the recent careless thoughts of a Harvard sophomore."

There is no sign the pandemic has prompted Big Tech to change its priorities. Silicon Valley has been involved in the pandemic response in three general areas: contact tracing, epidemic modelling, and public health communication. The industry has generally failed in the first and last of those. The tech titans have seen the crisis as another opportunity to expand operations without altering their underlying philosophy regarding commercialized data collection.

Europeans have been much more antagonistic than Americans toward consent-free data hoovering, but the pandemic crisis extended Big Tech's reach in the European Union. "Only a few European countries have publicly contested Apple and Google's involvement in digital contact tracing within the context of Big Tech companies threatening countries' capacity to regulate and retain control over their own digital infrastructures and data," according to researchers at the University of Oslo who studied Big Tech and the pandemic response. Public health agencies looking to use Apple and Google for contact tracing "have little if any choice but to accept the terms and conditions the companies impose" with respect to data ownership.

The French notably rejected the US tech companies' involvement in their contact tracing. Parliamentarians in Paris raised concerns about "making personal health data publicly available forever and allowing Big Tech and Wall Street to profit from them." The French people were instead asked to trust the state, which, through the national health care system, already maintains their health data.

Tiny Latvia also pushed back, accusing Big Tech of "dictating" European democracies' response to the pandemic. "In Latvia we wanted to harness smartphone technology for contact tracing. We ran into a Silicon Valley-built brick wall," Ieva Ilves, adviser to the Latvian president on information and digital policy, wrote in the *Guardian* in June 2020.

In past crises, Big Tech has donated data modeling in shows of corporate social responsibility—for example, during a cholera outbreak in Haiti. Big Data for Social Good, formed in Europe as the European Union was pushing back on data harvesting, is a project that donates data collection to humanitarian crises. The Oslo researchers took a skeptical view of those efforts: "That the data is offered pro bono during a public health crisis does not preclude their eventual monetization, however, and, according to our interlocutors, both Big Tech companies and telecom companies are devising mechanisms for future commercialization of their surplus data," they wrote.

Despite their vast reach, social media platforms have hardly racked up a stellar record in pandemic communications. Facebook has an obvious interest in promoting itself as a safe source of information, to counter its reputation as one of the great global purveyors of mis- and disinformation. A 2019 study termed Facebook's algorithms "a major threat to public health" because of their role in spreading misinformation.

Early in the crisis, Facebook chief Mark Zuckerberg gave the WHO a WhatsApp "chatbot" to assist the world body in sharing information with what was hoped would be at least two billion people. Two months after launch, it had only 12.6 million users, and the Oslo researchers "found no further information about its uptake since." WhatsApp refused to allow the chatbot to send users unsolicited notifications, and couldn't meet "the challenge of ensuring up-to-date information in a fast-changing context" or find answers to problems associated with communicating across linguistic and cultural lines.

The Oslo researchers concluded that "technologies ushered in during the Covid crisis may be reconfiguring the power balance between the public and private interests in ways that will far outlive the pandemic."

In the United States, few people are even asking these questions. The pandemic has simply pushed Americans ever faster and further into a no-touch, machine-dominated (and data-sucking) future, handing Silicon Valley titans what Naomi Klein calls a "Screen New Deal." Klein quotes a contactless parking app founder celebrating the new matrix thusly: "Humans are biohazards, machines are not."

THE HOME OF THE BRAVE

In the end, the body of America left bleeding at the end of Trump's presidency and the devastation of the eugenic pandemic marauding across a land without a unified medical response was a victim not only of the last four years but of decades of ascendant market capitalism.

The Trump administration didn't act as if it cared whether Americans got vaccinated or not. The promise to vaccinate twenty million Americans by the end of 2020 turned out to be a campaign slogan, nothing more. Money was being made in the chaos. Serving the public interest doesn't pay.

The Democrats came in and promptly passed a historic $1.9 trillion package they dubbed "American Rescue"—without a single vote of Republican support in the Senate. But nothing in the plan begins to address the structural problems in public health and policies with regard to the wealth inequality that made the pandemic so brutal for the poor and brown.

As Americans, we have agreed to live in a country that does not provide the safety net that citizens in every other country in the wealthy West take as a birthright. Many of us endure with the knowledge that we can lose our car, our life savings, and our home if we get really sick. We balance the cost of getting our teeth fixed or preventive surgery against the cost of college for our kids. Or we choose between paying the utility bills, paying the rent, and putting food on the table. As many as one hundred million Americans may have relied on food banks during the pandemic. The strain of this perpetual background anxiety on Americans' life and culture is palpable to anyone who has lived in countries with universal higher education and free national health care. The cost in terms of the burden on our economy may be incalculable—that is, will it put us into the history books of the future for the fastest decline of a leading nation in modern times?

It's a Washington axiom that we can't do anything to change traditional priorities. The cynicism is so deep, the passivity of the populace (until January 6, anyway) so entrenched, that deep recalculations of defense and public health spending are essentially off-limits to serious discussion. Politically savvy people think Medicare for All is a fantasy best left to "the squad" and "Bernie"—outliers in a political system controlled by money.

On February 10, 2020, the Trump administration submitted its budget proposal for 2021, including $740.5 billion for national security. That was a lot of billions to keep Americans safe from foreign foes when a nationless virus would soon kill half a million people. Those priorities have been boilerplate for decades. Between 1963 and 2017, US government discretionary spending on defense was never less than 48 percent of the total budget, and sometimes higher than 70 percent. Meanwhile spending on public health averaged between 3 and 6 percent annually.

Starting within weeks of the lockdown that began on March 11 with the closing of schools in New York, the big holes in the American public health care system and social safety net have become more and more obvious. No tests, and no way to trace the sick and their contacts. No protective gear for hospitals. Miles-long food lines. Sick people living paycheck to paycheck with no option but to continue to go to work, spreading the disease. Governors competing for equipment against other governors.

All this happened in the country that the experts—in one of their expert analyses just a few months prior to the lockdown—

had deemed to be *the most prepared* for a global pandemic of all the countries in the world.

The Trump regime's assault on federal agencies began in early 2017, but until March 2020, the immediate effect wasn't well understood. Now here came the proof: dismantling the federal government had made it incapable of responding to the urgent demands required of it during a pandemic.

As food lines grew, Congress deadlocked and calculated the meanest possible pittance to spend on the vast numbers of newly unemployed to help them pay for food and shelter. The discussion centered around this: Was more unemployment relief or direct government cash assistance going to keep lazy people from working? It sure smelled like socialism to cut a check for $1,200 for people who were doing nothing! When they finally passed the CARES Act, besides front-loading the legislation with bailouts for large companies, they chose to use an Econ. 101 word—"stimulus"—for the checks, so as not to alarm the flinty cranks.

Other rich nations were giving ten, twenty, or thirty times more in direct aid to their citizens than we were to keep them safe at home during the pandemic. Australia was subsidizing six million of its citizens' wages, Canada was paying its Covid-affected workers $2,000 a month, and Germany was subsidizing 60 percent of wages for employees who had reduced work hours due to the pandemic.

In the home of the brave, Americans would have to make do with $1,200 to last six months.

THE EUGENIC PANDEMIC

Since the end of Nazi Germany, it's been hard to find people who will stand up for the pseudo-science of eugenics outside of sweaty oompah band meeting rooms rented by Richard Spencer and David Duke. America's star fascists were briefly ascendant in 2017, enjoying a few moments of playing footsie with the mainstream during the early Trump years (Spencer even showed up, dapper, barbered, and in a suit, in Washington, DC, for Trump's inauguration). After the Charlottesville violence, and the resignation in disgust of Trump's entire business council, the Trump White House put public daylight between their movement and the "Heil Hitler" crowd. Not that they necessarily disagreed with the boys, or ever really severed ties (see: the Capitol insurrection).

They were just bad for business.

The Trump regime's handling of the pandemic was eugenic in effect if not in name. This is the awful legacy that we will all have to live with and remember, and use to inspire us to make real change.

By the end of 2020, more than half—58 percent—of people who had been in American hospitals with Covid were Black or Hispanic. And more than half of the nearly half a million dead—53 percent—were too. As a result, the discrepancy in life expectancy between Black and white populations in the United States grew to six years, a 46 percent increase from 2019 and the largest gap since 1998.

A very good CDC report on the racialized inequity in Covid sickness and death rates gets into the weeds to show how it has many causes. None of them are surprising, but the surprise may be just how many contributing factors there are that together amount to the crushing reality of racialized inequality in America today: discrimination in housing, discrimination in education, discrimination in health care, discrimination in criminal justice, discrimination in finance; limited access to health care and long-standing community distrust of health care providers; disproportionate minority presence in "essential" work, including at health care facilities, on farms, in factories, at grocery stores, and in public transportation; a tendency toward multigenerational households among minorities who are faced with housing discrimination and limited income to buy or to rent. That is not by any stretch a complete list. But it gives you an idea of the intersectionality of this reality, and how the different factors pile on and compound one another.

Once there was a vaccine, Black and Hispanic people—those most likely to get sick and die of Covid—were not at the front of the line to get it. Despite some early discussion of at least including the poor and brown among the high-risk groups to get first priority, that didn't happen. "In each population group, vaccine access should be prioritized for geographic areas identified through CDC's Social Vulnerability Index or another more specific index," the Advisory Committee on Immunization Practices advised the CDC in autumn 2020. The committee thought that the government should set aside portions of the first, limited supplies of the vaccine for Black communities hardest hit by the pandemic.

As the scale of the disparity became clear, Oxfam released a report blaming the American economic system for how the pandemic starved and killed the poor and brown while enriching the rich and white in America. "The worsening inequality crisis triggered by COVID-19 is fueled by an economic model that has allowed some of the world's largest corporations to funnel billions of dollars in profits to shareholders. At the same time, it has left low-wage workers and women to pay the price of the pandemic without social or financial protection."

WHAT AMERICANS HAVE HAD TO SETTLE FOR INSTEAD OF GOOD HEALTH CARE POLICY

In my decades covering politics, I have watched two Democratic Party efforts to create a national health care overhaul. The first, spearheaded by Hillary Clinton, was easily crushed by the insurance industry bent on keeping health care profiteers happy. The Obama administration's effort was more serious and was met with more serious opposition—including armed men menacing public hearings on the proposal.

The Affordable Care Act squeaked through, and the derisive name the right wing used for it—Obamacare—stuck as a badge of honor. It was far from perfect. But tens of millions of people were suddenly able to get health insurance, and for the first time Americans with preexisting conditions had a legal right to coverage.

In the decade since its passage, in a spectacle of shameless flintiness unrivalled in modern political history, Republicans filed dozens of lawsuits against Obamacare, trying every conceivable strategy to invalidate it.

Conservative think tanks like the Heritage Foundation poured tens of millions of dollars into research and legal strategy reports and staff hours aimed at crushing it. The Trump attack on the Affordable Care Act from inside the executive branch that was supposed to administer it increased the number of uninsured Americans by 2.3 million—and that was before the pandemic knocked millions more out of jobs that had provided them with health insurance. The rushed seating of Amy Coney Barrett was timed not only to the end of Trump's term but also to have her on the panel to hear a case that put the preexisting-conditions coverage of millions of Americans at risk.

Even with the pandemic as goad and exception, the profit-oriented model held fast. Medicare and Medicaid instituted a program to pay the Covid-related hospital bills of uninsured patients. But a study found that hospitals rarely informed the sick of this option.

The fear of a gigantic medical bill kept untold numbers of poor sick people home with Covid until it was too late to do anything for them. Others went to work sick and spread the virus. They had good reason to fear the bills: a still unknown number of large hospital systems continued to sue patients for unpaid medical debt through the pandemic.

In New York, for example, the nonprofit medical giant Northwell continued to file lawsuits against debtors as the pandemic knocked people off health insurance. "The Northwell lawsuits each sought an average of $1,700 in unpaid bills, plus large interest payments," according to a January 2021 report in the *New York Times*. "They hit teachers, construction workers, grocery store employees and others, including some who had lost work in the pandemic or gotten sick themselves."

The sheer helplessness of the poor against the menace of faceless creditors lurking behind every trip to the doctor or hospital added to the cruelty of pandemic unemployment, provoking private crises for untold millions of American families. The deaths of despair among America's poor and lower-middle class were already on the rise in the last decade. Covid accelerated that trend.

WHO WILL ASK RICH MEN TO SACRIFICE?

At the beginning of the pandemic, author and journalist Wade Davis wrote a scathing essay for *Rolling Stone* about Covid and "the end of America." He noted, correctly, that although the numbers of dead hadn't yet surpassed every other nation's, the pandemic extinguished the claim to American exceptionalism that the Trump regime sloganeered on. Buried in the essay is an important observation: that America in the 1950s was more like the Denmark of today than the America of today.

Tax rates in America in the mid-twentieth century for the wealthy went as high as 90 percent. Unions were strong. CEO salaries were only twenty times those of mid-management employees. American CEO pay has grown 1,000 percent since 1978; heads of companies today are paid, on average, 278 times what the typical American worker makes.

The pandemic has proven that market principles can't be applied to health care. The principles of supply and demand don't work when individuals will literally pay anything to stay alive, and when we are all made vulnerable by the vulnerabilities of any one of us. Wouldn't the people gasping for breath in the hallways of maxed-out California hospitals have signed over every dime they had in the bank to get the "cocktail" that was infused into Donald Trump and Rudy Giuliani? And won't we all feel—and be—safer once the least protected among us are safe?

Big Pharma executives and stockholders reaped a bonanza in the Operation Warp Speed public wealth transfer in pursuit of the vaccines and therapeutics, and this was business as usual. Between 2013 and 2017, the top five pharma companies—including Johnson & Johnson and Merck, recipients of federal Covid funds—all spent more on stock buybacks and dividends than they earned in profit, according to a study of Securities and Exchange Commission records published in *Salon*, helping themselves instead of benefitting the well-being of the public at large.

Economist William Lazonick has written about the effects of shareholder-centered drug and medical-care companies. "In the name of 'maximizing shareholder value' (MSV), pharmaceutical companies allocate the profits generated from high drug prices to massive repurchases, or buybacks, of their own corporate stock for the sole purpose of giving manipulative boosts to their stock prices," Lazonick wrote in a paper published in 2017. "Like no other sector, the pharmaceutical industry puts a spotlight on how the political economy of science is a matter of life and death."

Amazon founder Jeff Bezos doubled his wealth during this national disaster. One-seventh of his current hoard could end hunger in America. In September 2020, if Bezos had handed each of his 876,000 employees a $105,000 bonus, he would have been left with roughly as much wealth as he had at the start of the pandemic. In other words, the disparity is so great that there is literally no argument that further increasing the wealth of the super-wealthy provides any benefit whatsoever to the society at large. Whereas, to consider even for a moment the great benefit that broader and more equitable distribution of wealth could provide boggles the mind.

In December 2020, the total wealth of billionaires worldwide hit nearly $12 trillion—equivalent to the recovery spending of all the G20 governments put together, according to Oxfam. The ten richest people, including Bezos, Zuckerberg, and Tesla founder Elon Musk, had watched their combined fortunes rise $540 billion since March 2020. Ten percent of Americans own 80 percent of the stock market. The pandemic has made them all richer. After a terrifying dive in March and April, the market came roaring back and ended the year higher than ever—even while millions were out of work and poverty and hunger dramatically increased.

The rebounding stock markets and what Oxfam called America's "rigged economy" further exacerbated wealth inequality. Food lines grew. Evictions loomed.

Nothing about this obscene picture is accidental. It is a consequence of decades of a philosophy that came to prevail after Ronald Reagan's election. Somewhere around 1978, America began to devolve from a moderately synergistic nation where actor James Stewart's portrayal of Main Street banker George Bailey could serve as a universal role model into a society that openly celebrates greed and pure self-interest.

In some nations, the pandemic has prompted calls for an "excess profits tax" or onetime wealth tax. Argentina passed such a tax into existence, and as of this writing, British policy makers are discussing something similar. America had a wealth tax during World Wars I and II, and a wealth tax on corporations whose profits have soared due to the misfortune of the rest of the country, like Amazon, Zoom, and the drug maker Gilead, could help restore stability to economically shattered families and bring order to cities in apocalyptic freefall.

Oxfam has called for a Covid excess profits tax as a start to remedy the fact that seventeen of the top twenty-five US companies were expected to make more than $85 billion in "super-profits" for 2020 compared with 2019. The idea got instant pushback from the no-tax crowd. The Tax Foundation's Scott A. Hodge, for example, scoffed at the notion as "idealized" and claimed that the experience of previous generations had proven that such taxes were "difficult to administer, complicated to comply with, [and] undermined innovation."

THE WORLD WITHOUT US

We noticed it almost right away. In mid-March 2020, as the world shut down, there were way more stars in the night sky. The firmament was dusted with light, as if somehow shining a spotlight on the unfolding, unbelievable tragedy.

We thought we were imagining it. We were not.

Thanks to the lockdowns, emissions from aviation were down 50 percent from the prior year. The phenomenon was worldwide. The pandemic cut carbon emissions by 7 percent from 2019. Oil demand dropped by 435,000 barrels globally in the first three months of 2020, compared with the same period the year before. Coal-based power generation fell by a quarter to a third in India and China.

America had spurned the climate pact and now saw its modest goals, designed by hopeful men and women, as something of a global joke. But nature, in the form of the virus, was giving itself a reprieve from our abuse.

It's been a year. In the absence of my usual diversions—travel and the good society of friends—my misanthropic tendency, normally kept at bay, has resurfaced, directed both inwardly and outwardly. The smell of my own stale breath inside a sweaty mask disgusts me.

It's been a year. I live among the most privileged, richest, healthiest, safest humans in human history. We lost half a million of our citizens anyway. I twitch with silent irritation at the words on repeat in the podcasts and on TV and in the news stories: *Pain. Trauma. Healing.*

And the worst: *Self-care.*

The pandemic has not made us nicer or better. We are kernels of distrust. We are strangers to each other, loners. When we dare to meet friends or neighbors, there is always that initial, tense dance about whether or not to wear masks, even outdoors. We have learned to be suspicious in one another's presence. We make judgments on the varying degrees of precautionary care taken. We field or share suspicions about whose teen might have been out with friends the night before. We spew aspersions about who got the vaccine early and ask why and when and how.

Mostly we stay apart and alone. Waiting for something to change.

Out here where I am now, in the country, two hours from New York City, the roar of the occasional jet attracts our attention. We look up at the lone silver bird etched minuscule into the sky, watching with curiosity if not quite the awe of the cargo cult. Where have they gone, all those westward hourlies from LGA and JFK to Chicago and Denver and LAX? Will they ever come back? And if they do, will we board them?

Where do we want to go really?

And why?

CHAPTER 6

Uncertainty and Its Discontents

*"The best lack all conviction, while the worst are full of
passionate intensity."*

—W. B. YEATS

In the first edition of this book, I devoted a chapter to what
I called "Stranger Things," a taxonomy of conspiracy theories about the pandemic and the vaccines that proliferated
like kudzu—or like the SARS-CoV-2 virus itself. I cataloged
major theories and some outliers, from Trump's "it's a hoax"
to the anti-Chinese "Kung Flu" population control theory, to
the widespread belief that Bill Gates had somehow engineered
tracking microchips tiny enough to fit into hypodermic needles. I tried to identify the history and sources of these theories
and some of the motives—psychological, biological, political, financial—behind why so many people seemed to be so
attached to them.

My "Stranger Things" taxonomy has stood the test of time
and the march of events. But I did not predict that after another
year the crackpot infodemic would still be so persistent that vaccine misinformation and disinformation would have become an
integral element of our political and medical culture.

Today, a third of Americans, citizens of the richest nation on earth and availed of the best medical protection from the virus on earth—the mRNA platform vaccines—not only doubt the science of the virus and the vaccine but suspect the scientists of lying and, worse, maybe trying to kill them. One the nation's two major political parties disseminates and supports misinformation as part of its long game of Big Brotherish strategy to separate the public from fact-based reality.

Their most important collaborator is the most popular mass media outlet in the United States—Fox News. The vast misinformation network constructed by Rupert Murdoch and the owners of other nodes in the right-wing echo chamber is the foundation on which the US has achieved its shameful position as the nation with the highest number of Covid deaths in the developed world.

With virus variants eluding the vaccines, supply chains disrupted, and children around the globe having endured two years of disrupted education, it's become harder for public health officials anywhere to herd populations into forced faith in the power of science to get us "back to normal."

Americans' trust in the CDC and its ability to explain how to prevent and treat Covid-19 has continued to erode throughout the pandemic. As I write this, polling suggests that more than a quarter of Americans say they have no faith in the public health agency that used to be the gold standard for the world.

The revolt against vaccine mandates was global. The pandemic forced all governments to grapple with how to balance public health against civil liberties and personal choice. German, French, and British anti-vaccine protests erupted over the past year. Austria ordered the unvaccinated to stay inside their homes. Even South Korea, where a compliant population had followed orders and kept the virus under control for two years of the pandemic, was now revolting against mandatory vaccines for entry to grocery stores. Canada called a state of emergency as "Truckers for Freedom" clogged Ottawa and international entry points with parked rigs.

Americans, though, behaved more than just a wee bit crazier.

While anti-vax tennis star Novak Djokovic fought for his visa to the January 2022 Australian Open, self-described "Vaccine Police" leader Christopher Key, who calls the vaccine "the worst bioweapon I have ever seen," was driving around the United States with a flamethrower, advising people to cure Covid by drinking their own urine. "The antidote that we have seen now, and we have tons and tons of research, is urine therapy. OK, and I know to a lot of you this sounds crazy, but guys, God's given us everything we need," Key said in a video. "This has been around for centuries."

One of our two major political parties is calling life-saving vaccines totalitarian. During the pandemic Republican leaders not only encouraged risk, but increased it wherever they could by banning local mask mandates. The party has mainstreamed fringe thinking and quackery. Republicans latched on to the veterinary de-wormer, ivermectin, turning it into a code word for "liberty." No conspiracy theory is too wild. Former national security adviser Michael Flynn is only the most famous Republican preaching that Covid was created by George Soros, Bill Gates, and the WHO to make Donald Trump lose the 2020 election.

SCIENCE AND UNCERTAINTY

The lure of conspiracy theories and quack cures has deep roots in the human psyche. We are the most medically protected generation in human history. Science has given us tools to fight disease in ways unimaginable to the seventeenth-century Londoners facing bubonic plague in Daniel Defoe's chronicle, and even to Americans dealing with the Spanish flu a hundred years ago. Yet modern science communicators have not figured out how to break through something primeval in the human mind that prefers fiction, quackery, spirits, and conspiracy theory to facts when faced with a pandemic.

We are hardwired to be made anxious by uncertainty. And now that we have experts who actually do know how to transplant hearts, cure cancer, and fly man to the moon, we really don't like to be told, "We just don't know."

But not knowing—*uncertainty*, not certitude—is an integral part of modern science. The scientific process works like this: hypothesis, experiment, results, more questions, new hypothesis. Repeat. Repeat again. And again. And again.

Once the virus took hold, the demand for information in real time exploded. A steady supply of new but untested hypotheses flooded the academic world. Many were picked up and broadcast as certainties when they were still only hypotheses—by journalists on deadline, by presidents looking for quick cures. The virus was not airborne. Or was it? We did not need masks. Or, no wait, we did. Children were or were not spreading the virus. An old malaria cure definitely saved the sick. Or not? Nicotine seemed to protect smokers from severe Covid? (Yes, a study seemed to suggest this.)

Scientists in a position to reach the public, like those at the CDC, could barely keep up with the demand for information while sorting the wheat from the chaff in the supply of studies. And the scientific community set aside other research to concentrate their efforts on studying Covid, producing a tidal wave of new knowledge at an unprecedented speed. The WHO and CDC fumbled badly in the early days of the pandemic on the issue of masks. It took months for the scientific community to come to consensus on the airborne spread of the virus. While the experts went back and forth on their advice, hoarded hand sanitizer didn't seem to help anyone. Turned out, the virus traveled in invisible clouds from nose to nose. By the time consensus was reached and they told us to wear masks, the public recoiled at the prior months' long waffling and uncertainty of experts, that to some looked like lies, or ignorance.

"Since the beginning of this pandemic, it's been a piss-poor job, to say it in the nicest way," Dr. Syra Madad, an infectious disease epidemiologist at the Belfer Center for Science and International Affairs at Harvard, said of American public health communications.

Communications got even more challenging when the vaccine was rolled out. A significant minority of Americans remained stubbornly averse to being jabbed. Their concerns were not baseless. The history of vaccine development, going back to the cowpox, is one of tilts between success and sometimes deadly failure. Over time, numerous vaccines were invented, tested, and are now in mass use, preventing many childhood illnesses that used to kill or maim kids but that modern parents can't even pronounce. Sometimes vaccines have deadly side effects—the very first versions of a smallpox vaccine called variation sickened many and occasionally killed recipients, and a production problem during a 1955 mass vaccination effort against polio in the US killed dozens and sickened hundreds. Sometimes the severity of those side effects is only understood over time. Uncertainty is part of that process.

Vaccines, like most drugs, normally remain in evaluation

limbo for decades at the Food and Drug Administration (FDA) before reaching the public. But the pandemic was killing people and there was no time for years or decades of clinical trials and waiting periods. The FDA approved Covid vaccinations under so-called emergency use authorization.

In late 2020, the vaccines efficacy rates looked extremely promising based on a short series of small trials. Mass media heralded the coming shots as medical milestones and profiled their inventors as heroes. That wasn't wrong. But it wasn't the whole story either. Scientists had and still have no way of knowing for certain that the vaccines are utterly harmless for everyone over the long periods of time normally allotted for clinical study. No one wanted to hear or report too much on that, at first.

"You can see how in many aspects of society whether it's in politics, advertising, entertainment, sports, or even dating, simpler and more definitive messaging tends to resonate more with people regardless of whether the messaging is actually accurate," public health information expert Dr. Bruce Y. Lee told me. "Many people may falsely equate simpler, stronger, and overly confident statements with leadership, competence, and confidence. There has been what I've called the Tony Stark* portrayal of scientists on some TV shows and movies. People think that a scientist can just go into a self-funded lab alone for a few days and then magically emerge with a definitive solution that works. That's just not how science usually works."

The problem of communicating scientific uncertainty effectively to the public has been known and discussed for years. At a colloquium in 2018, Laura Helmuth, national editor of

---

* The brash and brilliant inventor in the Marvel Avengers franchise, whose alter ego is Iron Man.

health, science, and environment at the *Washington Post*, moderated a session on uncertainty in science communication. She talked about how difficult it is for journalists to explain science with limited space and in simple language, and how it can be tempting for them to simply leave out admonitions about uncertainty. "You have to pick your explanatory battles, and this is a battle that we often put off," said Helmuth.

INTO THE VOID

In 1999, David Dunning and Justin Kruger wrote a paper in which they claimed to have discovered a cognitive bias whereby people with limited knowledge or competence in a given intellectual or social domain greatly overestimate their own knowledge or competence in that domain relative to objective criteria or the knowledge of peers. Other scientists have since done studies that contradict this theory. But "the Dunning-Kruger effect" has cultural staying power as a way to explain the proliferation of overconfident ignoramuses in the two decades since it was first proposed. The fact that those two decades coincided with the growth of the World Wide Web probably has something to do with it.

"There are some people whose confidence outweighs their knowledge, and they're happy to say things which are wrong," Helen Jenkins, an infectious disease expert at Boston University, told the *New York Times*. "And then there are other people who probably have all the knowledge but keep quiet because they're scared of saying things, which is a shame as well, or just aren't good communicators."

Whether or not this is due to a cognitive phenomenon, a huge swath of Americans has been swayed by confident know-nothings when it comes to Covid. Rather than fading away as vaccines demonstrably lowered hospitalization and death rates, quack theories metastasized.

Conspiracy theorists have many advantages over truth tellers. Conspiracy theories are "self-sealing"—the exact opposite of science. Uncertainty is baked into the scientific process. New evidence must be considered and accounted for and hypotheses altered or rejected. The hallmark of conspiracy theories and pseudoscience is logical impenetrability. Believers will always use new or contrary evidence as further proof of the conspiracy itself.

Science is not infallible. Over the last decades, as super-computers have enabled or speeded up the collection of unprecedented quantities of data and remarkable advances have been made in the technology of medicine and its ability to fight disease, at the same time academics have worried about a "replication crisis," or what they call "irreproducibility." Papers get published with conclusions that aren't matched by subsequent experiments. One recent study found biomedical researchers expressed a decline in trust in the scientific enterprise, "in large part because the *quantity of new data* exceeds the field's ability to process it appropriately." In other words, the avalanche of new information might not just be confusing the public, but also clogging the pipelines of the greater brain trust in a way that has implications for the practice and reliability of modern biomedical science.

Conspiracy theories may assuage a basic human need for meaning and its relative, story. "A virus creates story-telling opportunities for debates about ethics that give us key information about characters. High stakes, a difficult problem and limited time—that's a solid recipe for fast-paced adventure," wrote Julia M. Wright, a Canadian literature and rhetoric professor. "This works well with American writer Joseph Campbell's hero-quest formula, widely used for script-writing, in which a hero, with helpers, must overcome a series of obstacles and opponents to eliminate a danger to his world."

Some of the major Covid conspiracy theories are literally lifted out of fiction. Mass vaccination campaigns to inject tracking microchips into millions of people was in season one of *The X-Files*. Akiva Goldsman, the screenwriter behind the Will Smith blockbuster *I Am Legend* felt compelled to tweet that the plot of his movie was all fiction. A *New York Times* report quoted one unnamed conspiracy theorist who said they feared the Covid vaccine because of the film, in which scientists botch an attempt to engineer the measles virus into a cancer cure, creating a new disease that turns most of humanity into zombies. "Oh. My. God. It's a movie. I made that up. It's. Not. Real," Goldsman tweeted.

Too late, Mr. Goldsman! Wright points out—and I agree—that simply fact-checking these fictions is probably not going to be enough to change people's minds. In real life, being fact-checked is humiliating. But for the fictional scientist-hero who stands up against the nefarious consensus, fact-checking simply proves that he or she "knows more than recognized experts."

The Covid-is-a-hoax cults and vaccine conspiracy theories demand belief—just like religions, which the pandemic-era mega-conspiracy cult Q Anon resembles. Conspiracy theories provide certainty just like God and his prophets. That's one reason why the unvaxxed and the most hard-core religious Americans overlap in the Venn diagram. Throughout the pandemic, many evangelical pastors watched their parishioners get sick or even die without pushing vaccinations, for fear of alienating them. Jackson Lahmeyer, a businessman and pastor of the three-hundred-member charismatic Sheridan church in Oklahoma, even sold tens of thousands of religious vaccine exemptions to anti-vaxxers.

"While trying to reason with a relative this past Christmas, I realized the microchip conspiracy theory—that COVID vaccines contain 'the mark of the beast' signaling alliance to Satan—also met powerful psychological needs," wrote Hannah Kim, a philosophy professor at Macalester and a former evangelical herself, in an essay on fiction and pandemic conspiracies. "One wants to be in control, chosen and special, 'awake' during End Times while others 'sleep.' . . . I see that cults and conspiracy theories get something right about our needs. We all need something or someone to tell us that we are in control or, at the very least, that we're OK. And for some people, that means embracing disinformation and false theories because they appear to offer answers or explain things we don't understand."

Besides the lures of quacks, fraudsters, movies, and fiction, partisan politics elevated pseudoscience and the anti-expertise sentiment for cynical gain during the pandemic. A significant number of conservatives believe that politics—liberal politics—drives scientific assessments of Covid's risk to human life and health. Same with the vaccines. That has led to a demographic phenomenon the *New York Times* data journalist David Leonhardt has christened "Red Covid." (More on that below.)

A year ago, Trump's politicization of science still had the capacity to shock. Today, it is accepted as a strategic tool of conservatives—and, for some, a way to make money.

One of the most effective vaccine misinformation mills under scrutiny is America's Frontline Doctors (AFLDS), connected with the secretive hard-right Council for National Policy. AFLDS was formed in spring 2020, and is one of many conservative organizations that supported efforts to reopen the economy while the pandemic was in its first deadly surge.

After the 2020 election, and after the vaccines became widely available, many anti-lockdown, pro-Trump organizations morphed into chaos agents to prevent the Democrats from looking successful. Some even made money on the side. By the end of 2021, AFLDS had referred more than a quarter of a million Americans to a quackery telemedicine enterprise called SpeakWithAnMD.com, operated by right-wing attack dog and former Roger Stone protégé Jerome Corsi. People forked over ninety dollars for their first call with "AFLDS-trained physicians" and then paid another sixty dollars per follow-up consultation. SpeakWithAnMD.com's "experts" then prescribed unproven coronavirus treatments, including ivermectin and hydroxychloroquine.

The so-called Frontline Doctors and Corsi's squadron of quackery are just two players in the disinformation game. Right-wing media sites such as OANN, Newsmax, and Fox have blasted doubt and denialism to hundreds of millions of Americans for two years now, calling the virus a hoax and equating vaccine and government public health mandates with totalitarianism. (Newsmax did temporarily suspend its star White House reporter for claiming that vaccines contain "Satanic trackers," an apparent bridge too far.)

Unfortunately, there is no accountability on the horizon for the behemoth at the center of this misinformation campaign. In late August, a Washington state appeals judge confirmed the dismissal of a consumer protection lawsuit against Fox News. The suit alleged that Fox talking heads—Sean Hannity, Tucker

Carlson, and Laura Ingraham, et al.—were liable for the lies they spread about Covid early in the pandemic. But the court responded that Fox had a First Amendment right to report on Covid as it did.

RED COVID

In the beginning, it infected the urban poor and their wealthier neighbors. It traveled silently among crowds, in high-rise elevators, around restaurants and theaters and subways. The first great surge killed New Yorkers in such numbers that forklifts were parked behind hospitals to haul away bodies for temporary storage.

The pandemic was originally a problem for Democrats in blue states. Presidential son-in-law Jared Kushner would reportedly take a pass on a full-fledged national testing strategy since the virus wasn't going to infect his father-in-law's supporters. But Americans living in suburban gated communities and on farms and ranches home on the range were not going to be spared. By summer and fall 2020, the virus was in diners and gas stations, laundromats, malls, schools, nursing homes, and especially hospitals. The cycles of death were soon neither red nor blue.

Then came the 2020 election, in which voters decisively rejected Donald Trump and his regime. Among his first acts in office, President Biden activated agencies and federal government powers that the anti-*gummint* forces in the previous administration had rejected. By spring, the vaccine was available nationwide and tens of millions were lining up to get it.

But then nothing went as planned. Trump's early politicization of the virus, dividing the country into alarmist liberal weenies and people who, like him, wouldn't let the virus "dominate" them, led to many tens of thousands more needless deaths.

The same people who believed the Big Lie about the election now also believed that the vaccines—developed at record speed thanks to Trump's decision to pour money into Big Pharma—were unnecessary at best and deadly at worst. Many clung to the cavalier attitude about the virus that their "real" president had modeled for them from the beginning.

Trump had greeted the incoming pandemic by comparing it to the flu, promising the virus would disappear "like a miracle" from America. Rather than disagree with their strongman, almost the entire Republican Party got in lockstep. Republican governors not only refused to require mask wearing, some enacted edicts outlawing local mask mandates.

Throughout 2020, the Covid attitude gap widened between Democrats and Republicans. By the time of the election, fewer than half of Republicans worried about Covid, while the vast majority of Democrats took the risks seriously. A year later, those same attitudes determined who got vaccinated. Nearly half of all Republicans still rejected the vaccine in late 2021.

These attitudes had deadly consequences. Interviewed in early 2021 on CNN, as Covid deaths approached half a million, Trump's own Covid czarina Dr. Deborah Birx said she believed all but the first 100,000 deaths were probably preventable. A Harvard study estimated that 135,000 unvaccinated Americans died unnecessarily in the last six months of 2021.

Then Red Covid swept the land in the form of new variants in the second half of 2021. The dead piled up in counties that had voted heavily for Trump.

AI data programs started to color-graph the phenomenon,

with politics on the horizontal line and deaths on the vertical. Red, dead. Blue, alive.

Bad optics, as Ivanka Trump would say.

As this trend grew more obvious, twinges of alarm emerged on the right. A Breitbart columnist trotted out a triple-axel conspiracy theory to explain the numbers. "If I wanted to use reverse psychology to convince people not to get a life-saving vaccination, I would do exactly what [Howard] Stern and the left are doing . . . I would bully and taunt and mock and ridicule you for not getting vaccinated, knowing the human response would be, *Hey, fuck you, I'm never getting vaccinated!*" wrote John Nolte. "No one wants to cave to a piece of shit like that, or a scumbag like Fauci, or any of the scumbags at CNNLOL, so we don't. And what's the result? They're all vaccinated, and we're not! And when you look at the numbers, the only numbers that matter, which is who's dying, it's overwhelmingly the unvaccinated who are dying, and they have just manipulated millions of their political enemies into the unvaccinated camp."

In fall 2021, the Trump team tried to backpedal the strategy of separating his supporters from the supposedly liberal life-saving science that would keep them alive. The RNC probably did an actuarial and realized all this death might hurt them at the midterms—even with gerrymandering and anti-democratic local laws in place.

So they trotted out the big guy to try to dial it back. In September 2021, in Dallas, on a tour with former Fox News commentator Bill O'Reilly, Trump was too late.

"Both the president and I are vaxxed," O'Reilly said, then looked over at Trump. "Did you get the booster?"

"Yes," Trump said.

The audience booed.

"Don't, don't, don't, don't, don't," Trump cried. "That's all right, it's a very tiny group over there."

FEAR OF THE UNKNOWN

Despite scientific advances that would have been unimaginable to those who lived through the last great pandemic a hundred years ago, the uncertainty that is a part of the scientific process tortures us. Scientific uncertainty and psychological uncertainty are not the same, of course. But the pandemic brought the two together.

Psychological uncertainty, according to recent research, might be the fundamental fear, the first fear that leads to all other fears. Primitive man, gazing out of the cave and into the cold dark, trying to make sense of a twig cracking. Wolf, enemy with a club, or a rabbit? Faced with uncertainty, the human brain instinctively conjures up monsters.

During the pandemic we endured isolation, job loss, financial insecurity, and watched as our children lost two years of education. But maybe the worst has been the anxiety born of the uncertainty of not knowing how or when the virus will come for us, and whether it will kill us or things will "get back to normal."

Researchers in neurology and psychology studying the effects of uncertainty on the brain say that open-ended uncertainty is one of the most insidious stressors we can experience as human beings. Fear of the unknown crushes our future-planning brains.

The brain's response to uncertainty—anxiety—is an evolutionary advantage, but too much of it is not good. Uncertainty disrupts both habitual and automatic mental processes that govern routine action, researchers believe. That disruption creates more conflict in the brain, which manifests as hypervigilance and emotional overreaction. "Uncertainty acts like rocket fuel for worry; it causes people to see threats everywhere they look, and at the same time it makes them more likely to react emotionally in response to those threats," the German science writer Markham Held has written.

For more than a year we have witnessed the effects of that rocket fuel all over America, in the myriad iPhone videos of people shrieking at store managers over masks in malls, of anti-maskers attacking flight attendants inside airplanes, of school board meetings transformed into mini-WWE spectacles, of men hurling racist epithets at store clerks who messed up their smoothies . . . and maybe even in the spittle-spewing faces of the people attacking the US Capitol with bats, flagpoles, and fists.

SORRY ANTI-VAXXER

On January 31, 2022, Dr. Anthony Fauci hopped on a call with the *New York Times* daily podcast. The *Times* wanted to know when, or whether, America might "get back to normal" or at least "enter the next phase." Omicron was on the wane. Hospital workers across the country seemed to be getting a break as the influx of mostly unvaccinated sick people in ICU beds was declining. Even blue state governors were flinging off the mask and lifting mandates.

The interviewer wanted to know, as we all have since the beginning of 2020: *What's going to happen next?*

Dr. Fauci had just endured two years fielding death threats

and right-wing caricature as the face of a global elite population-control scheme and its microchip-planting vaccine. Fox News had even promoted to a primetime slot an announcer who had urged people to "ambush" Fauci and "go in for the kill shot." The octogenarian's every utterance was routinely dissected by "Fauci-ouchie" anti-vaxxers and Covid-beat reporters alike.

So Fauci had learned to avoid making predictions. He wouldn't say when normal would come back or even what new normal would look like. He resisted going anywhere near *certainty*, to the frustration of the reporter and, probably, many listeners.

He did let slip a confession, though. He said he had abandoned hope of ever changing the minds of Americans refusing to get vaccinated. "I think, to be realistic, it's very clear that there is a hardcore group of people who do not want to get vaccinated," he said. The way forward, the way out of this dark place, he seemed to be saying, would be harder than it might have been because we would have to get there without the stubborn minority that refused to be vaccinated, depending only on people who believed in the science and got enough herd immunity to protect the science deniers.

At first Dr. Fauci's bleak assessment that tens of millions of Americans are in a state of impenetrable immunity to reason troubled me. But when I thought about it, the doctor's loss of faith in the power of science communication was no surprise. I too had lost faith in the power of political journalism to do what it was designed to do—educate the public and maintain the health of democracy. I lost that faith rather abruptly on an afternoon in summer 2018, in the middle of an arduous weeklong fact check on a long and complicated magazine cover article. I was overcome with the realization that whether we fact-checked our work or not, a large percentage of Americans now believed we were making it all up.

I probably should have noticed this much earlier, at least when the newly sworn-in president of the United States ordered his supporters to reject the "fake news" photographic and video evidence of his tiny inaugural crowd size and accept his claim that he had attracted the biggest crowd in inaugural history. It took me another year and a half to comprehend how the #fakenews movement, amplified by the most powerful megaphone on the planet, profoundly challenged all professions that deal in facts, including law and medicine. Like Fauci, in my own way, I too have come mostly to preach to the choir.

Volumes have been written on the failed dream of the internet ushering in a new age for democracy and free speech. The new agora of free expression was going to be an open arena where truth would "sally forth" and face off against lies, as John Milton put it in his essay *Areopagitica*, promoting unlicensed printing in the seventeenth century. Thirty years since the internet became a global commercial network, truth lies kicked and flailing on the floor of the digital square. Truth, it turns out, can be made malleable and is liable to be beaten to a pulp, mainly because the square is unpoliced and the crowds don't know how to judge information.

There is, though, a way back. Self-sealing conspiracy theories and attacks on "fake news" have one thing in common: they will never back down in the face of new information. While fact-based journalism shares something with real science: the willingness to revise, or to admit error. The easiest way to tell the difference between real and fake news, and between pseudo-science and real research, the sine qua non of all trustworthy information, it turns out, is the lowly, embarrassing correction.

As desperate as we are to avoid uncertainty, as instinctively as our amygdalae reject it, we should be wary of absolute certitude. Long before the publication of the Dunning-Kruger theory about the self-assurance of the uninformed, Voltaire wrote a simple axiom well worth remembering: "Judge a man by his questions, rather than his answers."

AUTHOR'S NOTE ON SOURCES AND METHODS

In order to understand the science, including the vaccine and the context in which it was developed, I started reading books on genetics, the history of vaccines, and the history of microbiology. I believe we can only truly understand and appreciate the race to the Covid vaccine if we understand the relatively short and utterly marvelous history of human understanding of pathogens and immunity, set against the long and terrible history of our ignorance.

Those books are listed below. Of them all, I found Paul de Kruif's lively history of the generations of experimenters and early modern scientists, written in 1926, both the most riveting and the most deeply moving. Arthur Allen's engaging history of vaccine science and Dr. Paul Offit's accessible dive into the challenges and triumphs of modern vaccine development were both invaluable and inspiring sources. Dr. Siddhartha Mukherjee's beautifully written book *The Gene: An Intimate History* was also a beacon for me.

To understand genetic medicine and the mRNA platform, I relied on my incredible research assistant, Vivian Zhong, PhD student in the bioengineering department at Stanford, who vetted the multitude of research papers and secondary source material available in the public domain and helped me select the best sources. Through that reading and with Vivian's help, I was able to visualize the chemical and biological processes and confidently describe them in what I hope is an accessible way. In addition to serving as my science teacher, Vivian early on reminded me of one of the chief reasons why this book is important. As she worked on one of the timelines, she emailed me, "I feel like I'm being pelted with WTFs all over again." In other words, to have to witness again the parade of willful negligence and cavalier missteps on the part of our government and the society at large.

And then there were the interviews I conducted, and the key insights they provided. I reached out to MIT chemical engineer Robert Langer, one of the founders of Moderna and an early experimenter in the long effort to get messenger RNA past the human immune system, who spoke with me about his work. Dr. Bruce Y. Lee of CUNY, a professor of public health policy and a health systems analyst, recounted how the pandemic preparedness community faced a political wall of inertia in the crucial early months. Moderna clinical trial participant Missy Peña, one of the first forty-five people in the word to receive an mRNA shot, shared her day-by-day recollections. Stanford microbiologist Dr. David Relman explained gain-of-function experiments and the Wuhan Institute of Virology lab-leak theory. Martha Louise Lincoln and Jessica Malaty Rivera helped me understand the anthropology of pandemics, our instinct for forgetting about them, and the challenges of science communication in an era of rampant mis- and disinformation.

—NB
New York, New York, 2021

AUTHOR INTERVIEWS

Robert Langer, January 10, 2021.
Bruce Y. Lee, January 13, 2021.
Martha Louise Lincoln, January 15, 2021.
Dr. Paul Offit, January 14, 2021.
Missy Peña, January 16, 2021.
David Relman, February 11, 2021.
Jessica Malaty Rivera, January 21, 2021.

BOOKS

Allen, Arthur. *Vaccine: The Controversial Story of Medicine's Greatest Lifesaver.* New York: W.W. Norton & Co., 2007.

Crick, Francis. *What Mad Pursuit: A Personal View of Scientific Discovery.* Alfred P. Sloan Foundation Series. New York: Basic Books, 1988.

Defoe, Daniel. *A Journal of the Plague Year.* Oxford: Oxford University Press, 1990.

de Kruif, Paul. *Microbe Hunters.* New York: Harcourt Brace, 1996.

Diamond, Jared M. *Guns, Germs, and Steel: The Fates of Human Societies.* New York: W.W. Norton & Co., 1997.

Grandin, Greg. *The End of the Myth: From the Frontier to the Border Wall in the Mind of America.* New York: Metropolitan Books, Henry Holt and Company, 2019.

Horton, Richard. *The COVID-19 Catastrophe: What's Gone Wrong and How to Stop It Happening Again.* Cambridge: Polity Press, 2020.

Kinzer, Stephen. *Poisoner in Chief: Sidney Gottlieb and the CIA Search for Mind Control.* New York: Henry Holt and Company, 2019.

Larson, Heidi. *Stuck: How Vaccine Rumors Start—And Why They Don't Go Away.* New York: Oxford University Press, 2020.

Manzoni, Alessandro. *The Betrothed*. London: Penguin Classics, 2016.

Mayer, Jane. *Dark Money: The Hidden History of the Billionaires behind the Rise of the Radical Right*. New York: Doubleday, 2016.

Mukherjee, Siddhartha. *The Gene: An Intimate History*. New York: Scribner, 2016.

Nichols, Thomas M. *The Death of Expertise: The Campaign against Established Knowledge and Why It Matters*. New York: Oxford University Press, 2017.

Offit, Paul A. *The Cutter Incident: How America's First Polio Vaccine Led to the Growing Vaccine Crisis*. New Haven: Yale University Press, 2005.

———. *Do You Believe in Magic? Vitamins, Supplements, and All Things Natural: A Look behind the Curtain*. New York: HarperCollins, 2014.

Oshinsky, David M. *Polio: An American Story*. Oxford: Oxford University Press, 2005.

Watson, James D., Andrew James Berry, and Kevin Davies. *DNA: The Story of the Genetic Revolution*. New York: Alfred A. Knopf, 2017.

Weisman, Alan. *The World without Us*. New York: Thomas Dunne Books/St. Martin's Press, 2007.

Zizek, Slavoj. *PANDEMIC! 2: Chronicles of a Time Lost*. New York: OR Books, 2021.

Zuboff, Shoshana. *The Age of Surveillance Capitalism: The Fight for the Future at the New Frontier of Power*. London: Profile Books, 2019.

SELECTED JOURNALS AND RESEARCH PAPERS

Himmelstein, David U., Steffie Woolhandler, Rebecca Cooney, Martin McKee, and Richard Horton. "The Lancet Commission on Public Policy and Health in the Trump Era." *The Lancet* 392, no.

10152 (September 2018): 993–95. https://doi.org/10.1016/S0140-6736(18)32171-8.

Koh, Howard K., Alan C. Geller, and Tyler J. VanderWeele. "Deaths From COVID-19." *JAMA*, December 17, 2020. https://doi.org/10.1001/jama.2020.25381.

Lapham's Quarterly, Summer 2020, Volume XIII, Number 3, "Epidemic."

Lazonick, William, Matt Hopkins, Ken Jacobson, Mustafa Erdem Sakinc, and Oner Tulum. "US Pharma's Financialized Business Model." *Institute for New Economic Thinking Working Paper Series*, no. 60 (July 13, 2017). https://doi.org/10.2139/ssrn.3035529.

National Academy of Sciences. *The Science of Science Communication III: Inspiring Novel Collaborations and Building Capacity: Proceedings of a Colloquium.* Washington, DC: The National Academies Press, 2018. https://doi.org/10.17226/24958.

Pardi, Norbert, Michael J. Hogan, Frederick W. Porter, and Drew Weissman. "MRNA Vaccines—A New Era in Vaccinology." *Nature Reviews Drug Discovery* 17, no. 4 (April 2018): 261–79. https://doi.org/10.1038/nrd.2017.243.

Siebert, Sabina, Laura M. Machesky, and Robert H. Insall. "Overflow in Science and Its Implications for Trust." *eLife* 4 e10825 (September 14, 2015). doi:10.7554/eLife.10825.

Storeng, Katerini Tagmatarchi, and Antoine de Bengy Puyvallée. "The Smartphone Pandemic: How Big Tech and Public Health Authorities Partner in the Digital Response to Covid-19." *Global Public Health*, February 18, 2021, 1–17. https://doi.org/10.1080/17441692.2021.1882530.

Wang, Fuzhou, Richard M. Kream, and George B. Stefano. "An Evidence Based Perspective on MRNA-SARS-CoV-2 Vaccine Development." *Medical Science Monitor* 26 (April 21, 2020). https://doi.org/10.12659/MSM.924700.

SELECTED JOURNALISM

Baker, Nicholson. "The Lab-Leak Hypothesis." *New York*, January 4, 2021. https://nymag.com/intelligencer/article/coronavirus-lab-escape-theory.html.

Bandler, James, Patricia Callahan, Sebastian Rotella, and Kirsten Berg. "Inside the Fall of the CDC." ProPublica. https://www.propublica.org/article/inside-the-fall-of-the-cdc?token=tg74b-8VQrqWdM-PFRUNWBD84ZpaGuM3h.

Eban, Katherine. "How Jared Kushner's Secret Testing Plan 'Went Poof into Thin Air.'" *Vanity Fair*, July 30, 2020. https://www.vanityfair.com/news/2020/07/how-jared-kushners-secret-testing-plan-went-poof-into-thin-air.

Green, Emma. "Health and Human Services and the Religious-Liberty War." *The Atlantic*, May 7, 2019. https://www.theatlantic.com/politics/archive/2019/05/hhs-trump-religious-freedom/588697/.

Piller, Charles. "The Inside Story of How Trump's COVID-19 Coordinator Undermined the World's Top Health Agency." *Science*, October 14, 2020. https://www.sciencemag.org/news/2020/10/inside-story-how-trumps-covid-19-coordinator-undermined-cdc.

Reuters. "Timeline—In His Own Words: Trump and the Coronavirus." October 3, 2020. https://www.reuters.com/article/us-health-coronavirus-usa-trump-comments-idUKKBN26N0U5.

Shear, Michael D., Noah Weiland, Eric Lipton, Maggie Haberman, and David E. Sanger. "Inside Trump's Failure: The Rush to Abandon Leadership Role on the Virus." *The New York Times*, July 18, 2020. https://www.nytimes.com/2020/07/18/us/politics/trump-coronavirus-response-failure-leadership.html.

Weiland, Noah. "'Like a Hand Grasping': Trump Appointees Describe the Crushing of the C.D.C." *The New York Times*, December 16, 2020. https://www.nytimes.com/2020/12/16/us/politics/cdc-trump.html.

Weiland, Noah, Sheryl Gay Stolberg, and Abby Goodnough. "Political Appointees Meddled in C.D.C.'s 'Holiest of the Holy' Health Reports." *The New York Times*, September 12, 2020. https://www.nytimes.com/2020/09/12/us/politics/trump-coronavirus-politics-cdc.html.

VIDEOS AND PODCASTS

"Alex Jones Warned of Covert Operation to Cull the Elderly." https://banned.video/watch?id=5f3c2260df77c4044ee7a70f.

"Coronavirus Pandemic Is Now an (Open Source) Biological Weapon." https://banned.video/watch?id=5e3784aa113ab20016b1a504.

"In the Groves of Misinformation: Making Sense #233." https://sam-harris.org/podcasts/233-groves-misinformation/.

"President Trump Visits Centers for Disease Control and Prevention." https://www.c-span.org/video/?470138-1/cdc-send-million-coronavi-rus-testing-kits-week.

"We Need to Talk About Covid, Part 2: A Conversation with Dr. Fauci." https://www.nytimes.com/2022/01/31/podcasts/the-daily/we-need-to-talk-about-covid-part-2-a-conversation-with-dr-fauci.html.

Vernon Coleman on the "Covid Hoax." https://brandnewtube.com/@DrVernonColeman.

DOCUMENTS

Warren, Elizabeth, and Richard Blumenthal. "Warren and Blumenthal to Medical Equipment Wholesalers: Explain Your Role in the Jared Kush-ner-Led 'Project Air Bridge' That Failed to Provide Critical Supplies for States' COVID-19 Responses." April 27, 2020. https://www.warren.senate.gov/oversight/letters/warren-and-blumenthal-to-medical-equipment-wholesalers-explain-your-role-in-the-jared-kushner-led-project-air-bridge-that-failed-to-to-provide-critical-supplies-for-states-covid-19-responses.

Warren, Elizabeth, Charles Schumer, and Richard Blumenthal. "Letter to PRAC Re Project Airbridge." June 8, 2020. https://www.warren.senate.gov/imo/media/doc/Letter%20to%20PRAC%20re%20project%20airbridge%202020.06.pdf.

ABOUT THE AUTHOR

Nina Burleigh is a journalist and author of six prior books, including most recently *The Trump Women: Part of the Deal* and the *New York Times* bestseller *The Fatal Gift of Beauty: The Italian Trials of Amanda Knox*, of which Tim Egan wrote: "Clear-eyed, sweeping, honest and tough . . . sets a standard that any of the other chroniclers of this tale have yet to meet. This is what long-form journalism is all about." She most recently covered America under Donald Trump as national politics correspondent at *Newsweek*. She got her start in journalism covering the Illinois Statehouse in Springfield, Illinois, and is a fellow of the Explorers Club who has covered stories on six continents.

Burleigh's writing has appeared in *Rolling Stone, The New Yorker, Time, New York, The New York Times Magazine, Slate* and *Bustle*. She has appeared on *Real Time with Bill Maher, Good Morning America, Nightline, The Today Show, 48 Hours,* on MSNBC, CNN, C-SPAN, NPR, in numerous documentaries, podcasts, and radio programs. A former judge for the J. Anthony Lukas prize for nonfiction, Burleigh is an adjunct professor at NYU's Arthur L. Carter Journalism Institute. Her work has been cited in hundreds of scholarly articles.